New Directions in
Health Education

New Directions in Health Education

School Health Education and the Community in Western Europe and the United States

Edited by

George Campbell

The Falmer Press

(A member of the Taylor & Francis Group)

London and Philadelphia

UK	The Falmer Press, Falmer House, Barcombe, Lewes, East Sussex, BN8 5DL
USA	The Falmer Press, Taylor & Francis Inc., 242 Cherry Street, Philadelphia, PA 19106-1906

Copyright © Selection and editorial material G. Campbell 1985

First published 1985

Library of Congress Cataloging in Publication Data

Main entry under title:

New directions in health education.

Bibliography: p.
Includes index.
1. School hygiene—Europe—Addresses, essays, lectures.
2. Health education—Europe—Addresses, essays, lectures.
3. Community and school—Europe—Addresses, essays, lectures.   4. School hygiene—United States—Addresses, essays, lectures.   5. Health education—United States—Addresses, essays, lectures.   6. Community and school—United States—Addresses, essays, lectures.
I. Campbell, George, BSc, MA, DipEd.
LB3409.E85N48   1984   371.7′094   84-18718
ISBN 0-905273-58-3
ISBN 0-905273-57-5 (pbk.)

Typeset in 10½/12 Plantin by
Imago Publishing Ltd, Thame, Oxon.

Printed in Great Britain by Taylor & Francis (Printers) Ltd, Basingstoke

Contents

Contents

Acknowledgements

I wish to express my thanks firstly to the University of Southampton Committee for Advanced Studies which funded my extended visit to Western Europe from which the idea grew for an International Seminar on School Health Education. Secondly, my thanks to the British Council for financing the travel of several colleagues from abroad for the Seminar. Thirdly, my thanks to those colleagues who supported the idea and the subsequent work but whose names do not appear in the text; principally Professor Dr K. Vuylsteek of the University of Gent, Professor K. Ostyn of the University of Leuven, Dr Rosmarie Erbon of the Federal Centre of Health Education in Cologne, Dr Jos v. Hameron of The Netherlands National Centre for Health Education and Professor Peter Kelly, Dean of the Faculty of Educational Studies, University of Southampton.

I am deeply indebted to the following colleagues for their contribution to the success of the Seminar and subsequently at the editorial stage for their advice, comment, constructive criticism and sub-editing: Pat Christmas, Eugene Donoghue, Martin Evans, Peter Farley, Mary Holmes, Heather Hyde, Stanley Mitchell, Lewis Slack, Trefor Williams and Charles Wise. Finally, my thanks to Jill Anderson who assisted in the running of the Seminar, and Annette Bailey who typed the manuscript.

Introduction: New Directions in Health Education

The last ten years have seen greater developments in health education in school and community than at any period in the past; yet much still remains to be done. The most marked progress has been in the countries of Western Europe, in particular the United Kingdom, and in North America. Within health education generally the greatest concentration of activity has been in school health education where a guaranteed audience is provided over an average ten-year period of compulsory attendance. Where the emphasis has been on primary school health education this has been associated with the laying down of secure foundations early in life upon which, hopefully, can be built positive attitudes to health and wise decisions later on. While progress has been good, its distribution is uneven and many schools in the countries referred to above remain little affected by recent developments.

Behind the upward trend lies a declining belief in the high technology aspects of curative medicine and a corresponding strengthening belief in the preventive. However, belief is not necessarily followed by action, and progress towards good health via prevention remains patchy and generally slow. A clearer understanding of many of the causes of ill-health has now . emerged, but its application in planned programmes of health education and health promotion has been limited and has only begun to filter through to the public consciousness. The so-called 'diseases of civilization': cancer from environmental causes; heart disease and respiratory disease both associated with smoking, diet and lifestyle; mental illness associated with alcoholism and drug-taking; and road accidents, account for an increasing proportion of human suffering, serious illness and death in the western countries. Yet the enthusiasm of governments to initiate policies and programmes of legislation, information or education calculated to reduce the level of suffering and positively promote good health remains obstinately low. When individual cases are scrutinized government reluctance is more readily understood. For example, although the pressures for legislation against smoking in public places are considerable, governments may be unwilling to legislate because of the fear of loss of a major source of revenue. Every country in Western Europe has experienced a major increase in cigarette smoking since the Second World War and governments have become increasingly dependent upon the tobacco taxes which are raised. In the field of health education, governments may baulk at the high cost of national curricular innovations where evaluation is inconclusive and longer-term results may be in doubt. In this respect health education suffers because of being a part of education which is itself notoriously difficult to measure and evaluate. These issues repeat themselves at local level where local authorities may be reluctant to embark on a curricular innovation for all of their schools because of the cost of materials and teacher time-off for in-service training.

It is not only government which may be slow to initiate new developments. Professional bodies, particularly influential ones such as doctors and teachers, are frequently unable to agree firm policies because of lack of conclusive evidence. For the medical profession, the nature of the association between diet and coronary heart disease and for the teaching profession the effectiveness of school programmes of education about smoking are but two of many examples.

Many national organizations in the western countries have confronted these issues and more, attempting to resolve them as a first step to recommending appropriate action. At an international level organizations such as the World Health Organization (WHO) have widened debate, increased the scale of involvement and begun to wield a stronger influence generally. Since the 1960s the WHO Regional Office for Europe has conducted a series of international seminars on major health issues. One held at Gent, Belgium in 1980[1] examined in considerable detail the constraints surrounding 'education for health of schoolchildren and parents' and made these specific recommendations, all of which reflect acute school-community concerns:

1   Consideration should be given to the development of a theoretical model which would serve to illustrate the dynamic relationship between different elements and components in society which interact to determine the quality, nature and persistence of constraints affecting education for health.
2   All necessary measures should be taken to create openness and dialogue between schools and their communities.
3   Investment should be concentrated on integrating the principles of health education into the preparation and training of all professional groups involved with community work.

The common factor in all three recommendations is a recognition of the importance of the school-community relationship and the difficulties surrounding it.

The purpose of this volume is to study the interface between school and community to assist in the identification of policies, strategies and methods likely to achieve better planned and coordinated health education through the priorities recommended above. The papers which comprise the volume are grouped under appropriate key headings and together form a critical review of thinking and action on the part of leading health educators in Western Europe and the United States. All the papers are original, were written specifically on the school-community interface theme and refer to current or recent work in a particular country. The preoccupation with issues in a Western European and United States context is due solely to their experience of common problems in health and health education which are the result of common influences in their respective cultures.

Part 1 examines the nature of the constraints confronting those who would promote school-community interaction in school health education. Part 2 examines policies, strategies and methods of overcoming the constraints. Part 3 examines the special contribution of professional training, initial and in-service, to the progress of school health education. Part 4 is a selective study of post-1981 developments in the named countries, with the exception of the paper by Maes. Part 5 simply sets out a record of post-1981 developments in the United Kingdom, because of the widespread interest displayed in the new directions being taken there. Since ultimately innovations depend upon regional and local initiatives and support, an outline of some developments at regional and local levels is included in addition to the more widely known national developments.

The first eight chapters[2] were originally presented as papers at the International Seminar on School Health Education held at the University of Southampton in 1981. Detailed discussions of them, based on reports from working groups, are set out in the Appendix. In these discussions the ideas presented within each paper are reviewed, extended and exemplified, and new directions are charted.

Note

1 WHO Symposium on Constraints in Education for the Health of Schoolchildren and Parents, Gent, 29 September–3 October 1980.
2 These comprise all papers upto and including Maes.

Part 1. Understanding the Constraints on School-Community Interaction

Introduction

Trefor Williams and George Campbell present joint chapters on the topic, 'Towards a Model of School-Community Interaction', Williams taking a school standpoint, Campbell a community standpoint, both essentially raising and clarifying issues.

Williams identifies three basic concepts which can serve to provide a context for a model of school and community interaction:

1 *The Health Career* which provides a means of reviewing the many influences which help shape values, attitudes, skills and behaviour having a bearing upon health.

2 *The Spiral Curriculum* which has largely been used in the context of the school curriculum. Briefly it is based upon the belief that if certain ideas or concepts are valued by a community/society they can be taught and are relevant to every age group. It is arguable that what is true for the school curriculum is also highly relevant for the school-community interface.

3 *Coordination*, a concept which has been explored at some depth by the Schools Council Health Education Project (SCHEP) as a means of harnessing the human and material resources available in a school to the task of planning and implementing a programme of health education for its pupils.

The concepts of *Health Career* and *Spiral Curriculum* as discussed in the context of school-community interaction imply — indeed demand — a high level of coordination of the skills and knowledge possessed by many professional groups. They imply the drawing together of various professions which are not normally in close communication with each other and which sometimes do not even understand each other's functions. Who is to take responsibility for such coordination — should the locus for it be inside or outside the school, should the initiative rest with education or health authorities?

The paper concludes by considering some of the factors which might influence the nature and level of coordination.

Campbell's chapter examines the obstacles to 'the common understanding', in particular the boundary problems between school and community which prevent or limit productive collaboration. These are interpreted as differences in perception of critical issues: what health education is, and what are the necessary tasks, roles and skills required to achieve its goals. Examples of local empirical work are drawn upon to indicate the importance of task-centred activities as a means of developing interagency understanding and, ultimately, cooperative action. The emergence of key management principles is noted, and the paper concludes with a discussion of the 'coordination' role.

A discussion of the points raised in these chapters is set out in the Appendix pp. 211–3.

Health Education and the School-Community Interface: Towards a Model of School-Community Interaction:
I: A School View

Trefor Williams

Because the health related behaviours of young people are largely practised outside the classroom in the wider school and community environment it follows that the teaching of health education should seek to link these areas of operation more closely together. For example, if as a matter of principle a school accepts the importance of teaching about human and personal relationships, this will have implications for its own organization, structure and internal relationships. If what is learned in the classroom is not seen to be supported in practice by the school environment it will have little validity in the eyes of the students. Such teaching and learning will also need to demonstrate the validity of the principle to the lives of people in the wider community if it is to hold credence as an important and relevant area of human concern.

This issue of school and community interface emerged as an area of central importance in the 1980 World Health Organization European Region Symposium held in Gent, Belgium. The Symposium, 'Constraints in the Education for Health of Schoolchildren and Parents', brought together representatives from sixteen European countries for five days of intensive discussion. The Summary Report of the Symposium offered three specific recommendations:

1 Consideration should be given to the development of a theoretical model which would serve to illustrate the dynamic relationship between different elements and components in society which interact to determine the quantity, nature and persistence of constraints affecting education for health.

2 All necessary measures should be taken to create openness and dialogue between schools and their communities.

3 Investment should be concentrated on integrating the principles of health education into the preparation and training of all professional groups involved with community work.

Trefor Williams (UK)

The present Seminar in Southampton partly arises out of the challenge implicit in these three recommendations — a challenge, it is felt, which needs to be taken up and developed by a continuing and dynamic dialogue, research and action in Europe and in other countries. The purpose of this

Figure 1.   Health Education

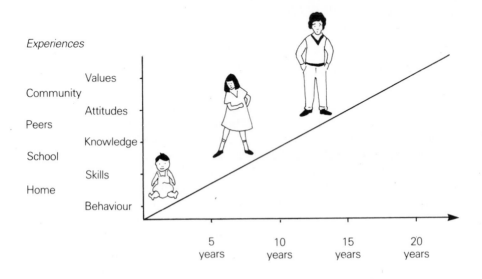

Development sequence — age

Health Education   (general sense)
'All those experiences from which we derive *knowledge, attitudes, values* and *skills* which influence health behaviour' — *synonymous with process of socialization*

Health Education   (specific sense)
'Those planned experiences, at home, school or community from which knowledge, skills, insights, attitudes and behaviour relevant to personal and community health are established.'

School Health Education
'Those planned experiences, both formal and informal, which contribute to the establishment of knowledge, skills, attitudes and values and which help an individual make choices and decisions relevant to health and well-being.'

and the following chapter is to begin this dialogue by offering some basic ideas and concepts for consideration. This contribution is intended to serve as a frame of reference for a model of school-community interaction and is based upon several concepts which have become, for me, basic and essential to a personal construct of health education.

The first concept is that of the *health career line* which provides an outline review of the chief influences on the health behaviour of individuals in a given community or society (see Figure 1). For the purpose of this paper the term 'community' refers to a social group of people, subjected to the same general laws and customs and also to certain categories of experiences, referred to as its culture, which influence thinking, behaviour and lifestyle. It is possible, for example, to demonstrate the influences exerted by the home, friends and community upon the emergent smoking behaviour of young people or upon attitudes to alcohol. It is possible to view the resultant

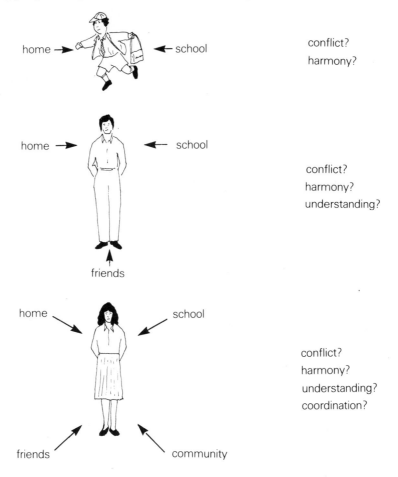

Figure 2. *The Timing of Various Social influences*

behaviour as a product of the interaction between a growing/developing personality and these social influences. It is also possible to take snap shots of the possible dominant influences at any one time, so that, for example, when a child has just started school it seems reasonable to postulate the main influences as stemming from home and school, while later during pre-pubescence the influence of friends can be added. Similarly at mid/late adolescence there will be the added influence of the community environment and possibly the work situation (see Figure 2).

The important question is *what* messages about health or health behaviour are transmitted both formally and informally by each of these influences. Are the formal and informal messages stemming from a single influence contradictory or complementary? Are the messages coming from the major influences complementary or contradictory? Are there ways in which the various categories of health messages could be recognized, classified and coordinated? Are we indeed confident that we know what the messages should be at any one stage of development?

The second concept is that of the *spiral curriculum* which is well-known and understood in the context of the school. I feel that it has application also to school-community interaction. The basic idea is straightforward: if an idea or concept is thought important enough and is valued by a community

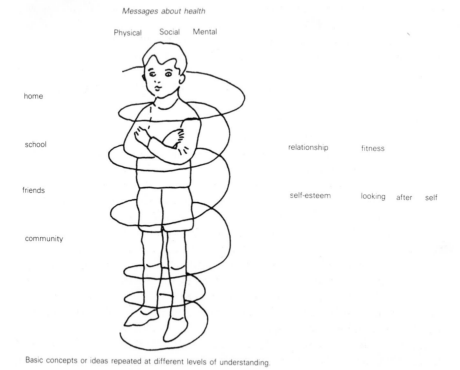

Basic concepts or ideas repeated at different levels of understanding.

Figure 3. The Spiral Curriculum

then it is possible to relate it to any level of understanding from early childhood to late adolescence and beyond. Once a decision has been taken concerning the concept it is feasible to repeat it at an increasing level of complexity commensurate with the level of understanding and of relevance to the recipients. In this way the same concept can be considered and related to the needs and aspirations of all groups — including children and young people — in the community (see Figure 3).

The mechanism by which the spiral curriculum operates in the community is largely through socialization where what is 'valuable' or 'permissible' is made clear through a system of formal and informal messages reinforced by rewards, punishments and other sanctions. The spiral curriculum operates in schools by the choosing of areas of study which are seen to be 'worthwhile' educationally. These can be divided into the two facets of school life, generally referred to as the 'academic' and the 'pastoral'. 'Academic' refers here to those traditional subject areas of the school curriculum which form the 'backbone' of teaching in the school. 'Pastoral' is used as an all-embracing term for those areas of school life which encourage the social and personal development of pupils. They are not mutually exclusive — indeed they ought, as Hamblin argues, to be seen as partners in the same educational process. Marland points out that where they are treated as separate parts of the life of a school the 'pastoral' is in danger of being seen as inferior by both staff and pupils. In terms of the operation of the spiral curriculum for pastoral care/health education it is then first necessary for the school itself to value this area of work sufficiently to accord it an important place in the curriculum. Secondly, it would be necessary for a school to think through the real implication of this for the way in which the curriculum, both in terms of content and methods of teaching, is organized for its pupils.

What, in terms of the spiral curriculum which in theory can link schools to the community, are the health messages or concepts which are valued or seen as educationally worthwhile? Is it possible to establish some basic concepts related to health which can be used as focal or starting points for the community-school spiral curriculum? One of the obstacles to reaching such basic concepts is the difficulty in establishing a common understanding, amongst those professional and lay persons involved, of health and health education; a common understanding which could provide a sense of common purpose. There have been attempts to make a conceptual analysis of the health education field, notably that of the American School Health Education Study which produced its excellent *A Conceptual Approach to Curricular Design* in the 1960s and which has been a wellspring of other significant developments both in the United States and elsewhere. The concepts needed as a base line for a shared understanding must, however, be related to ideas implicit in the professional training and work of community workers and teachers and must also make sense to parents and other involved lay persons.

For a school-community model I find it expedient to use three basic concepts:

1 Relationships   — both personal and interpersonal;
2 Self-management — caring for and looking after self;
3 Community   — caring for and interacting with the environment.

Each of these will need to be developed into sub-concepts relating to the level of understanding and development of the recipients. I am suggesting that the three concepts could form a common base line for school-community interaction (see Figure 4).

The third concept I wish to explore is that of *coordination*. It is possible to argue that health education can be seen *primarily* as an orchestration of the many influences to which individuals are exposed. Indeed, given the broad-based nature of health education itself it is difficult to conceive of how

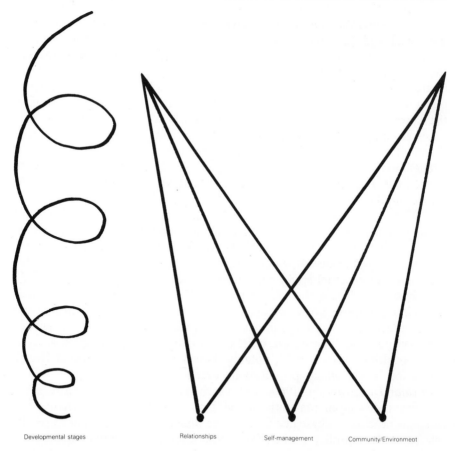

Developmental stages   Relationships   Self-management   Community/Environment

Figure 4.   Three Basic Concepts of Health Education Related to the Spiral Curriculum and How They Interrelate.

a programme of health education could succeed in either school or community without a degree of cooperation and coordination between the personnel and agencies involved.

The later of two Schools Council Projects in Health Education — concerning secondary schools — recognized the importance of a coordinated approach to health education across the curriculum. At a very basic level, for example, the health teaching which occurs across the many subject areas can be made more effective by coordinating their content and timing. From the pupils' point of view it is important to ensure that the many messages stemming from various subject areas are consistent with each other and provide coherent, clear and relevant health education messages. Of course, much more than this is involved in a properly planned and coordinated programme of health education, but it does demonstrate how the quality of what is provided can be enhanced considerably by making more effective what already exists (see Figure 5). In the same way that coordination implies

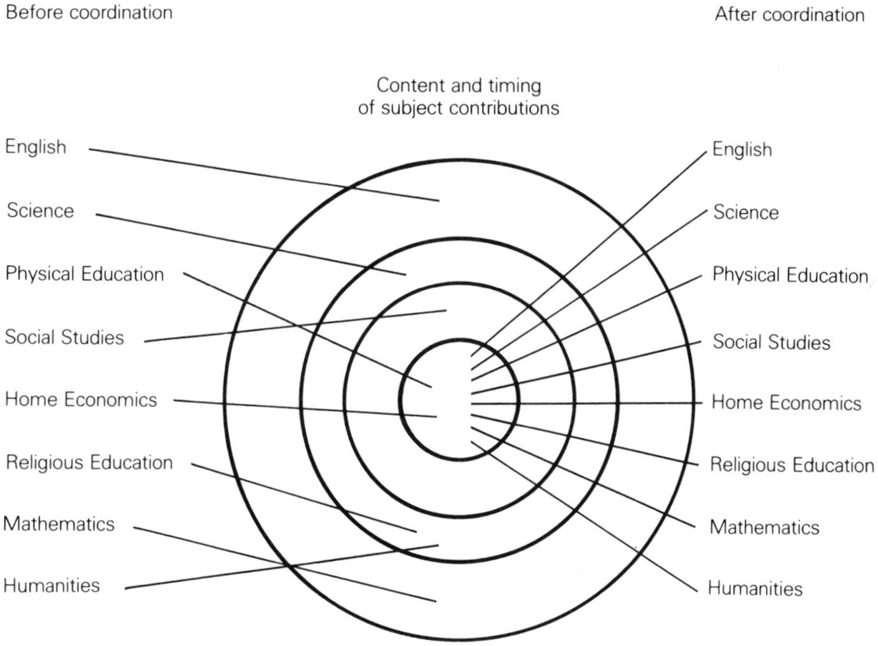

Before coordination   After coordination

Content and timing
of subject contributions

English   English

Science   Science

Physical Education   Physical Education

Social Studies   Social Studies

Home Economics   Home Economics

Religious Education   Religious Education

Mathematics   Mathematics

Humanities   Humanities

The 'bullseye' represents the pupil's perception of what has been learned in terms of coherence and relevance.

Figure 5.   *Coordination of Health Education across the Curriculum*

Trefor Williams (UK)

a cross-curriculum consideration for schools, so too it implies a consideration of cross-professional and agency interaction between school and community. Again, from the pupils' perspective it is important to demonstrate that the values, attitudes, skills and behaviour which are considered important in the school are demonstrably important to and in the community — and vice versa. It is difficult if not impossible to ensure such coherence without consultation between school and community agencies and, as important, without some kind of community dimension or base to the health education curriculum itself. This has implications not only for *what* learning experiences are offered to pupils but also for *how* and *where* and *by whom* they are offered. In brief, a school needs to make good use of the human and other resources available to it not only from within its own boundaries but also from the community itself (see Figure 6).

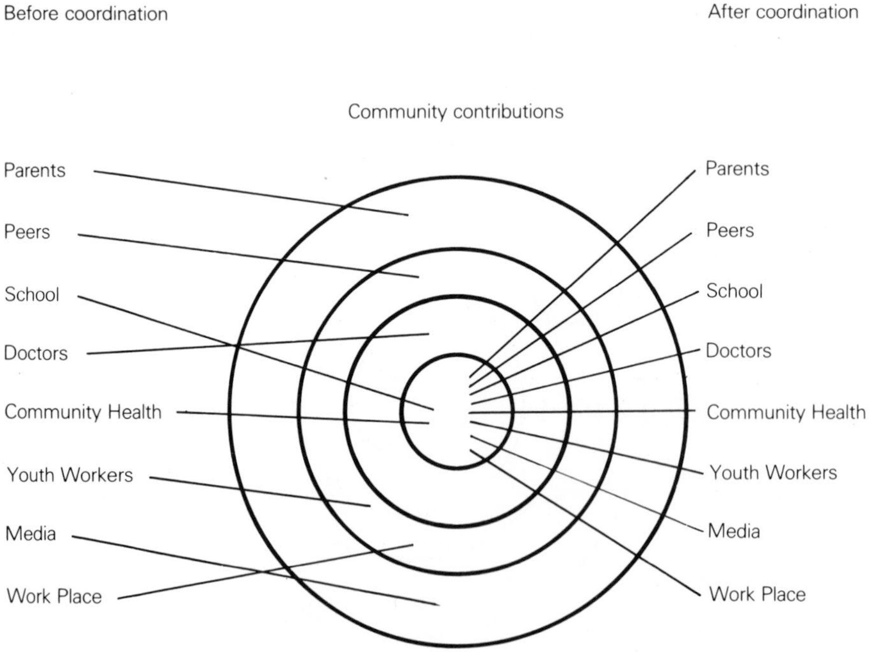

The 'bullseye' represents the degree of coordination among various community agencies resulting in a coherent policy.

Figure 6. *Health Education and the Community*

14

Is there a base of common purpose and concern from which a *shared*, *unified* and *coordinated* action might result? I believe that there is. The major obstacle to such a measure of coordination is the lack of a single agency or person to take such an initiative. From whence should such an initiative come? From Education? From Health Services? To be effective on a wide scale, national agencies must be involved, particularly if the initial and in-service training of a variety of professional groups is to be influenced (see Figure 7). In the short term, it is likely that local initiatives will give the best return for effort. Several such efforts come to mind:

1   the report by Dr Sennerfeldt, Chief Medical Officer for Schools, Sweden, of an experiment of two schools making use of the resources already existing in the school and community;

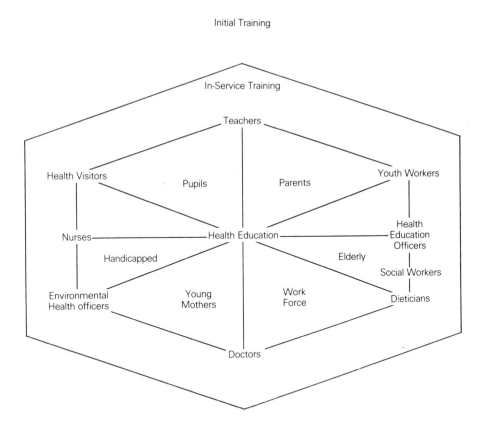

Figure 7.   A Web of Interaction to Bring About a Coordinated Community Policy Involving Both Pre-Service and In-Service Training

2 George Campbell's work in Hampshire (which is discussed in the next chapter);
3 the larger-scale work of Helen Nowlis in the United States.

While the initiative for each of these projects comes from outside the school, each has struck a responsive chord in the school concerned. It is obvious that at least two *levels* of coordination are involved: that concerned with *coordination* within the school itself and that of managing the coordination and negotiations between school and community agencies.

There are several questions to ponder:

1 Are there persons who could take-on the role of School Coordinator?
2 What knowledge and skills would they need to carry out such a task?
3 Are there persons available to assume the role of Community Coordinator?
4 What special skills would they require?
5 How are such persons to be trained?

Health Education and the School-Community Interface: Towards a Model of School-Community Interaction:
II: A Community View

George Campbell

Boundary Problems between School and Community

In the United Kingdom in recent years we have, in national and local school curriculum and staff development policies, attempted to start from where the pupils and teachers are. In doing so we have come into conflict with boundary problems of different kinds, boundaries which mark off where one teacher's responsibility ends and another's begins; boundaries which may be demarcated territorially, clearly, for all to see, or which may not, but simply exist in the minds of individuals as social or psychological barriers, and never revealed until a dispute arises.

The school-community interface marks a boundary in the same way that a frontier demarcates two nations, with their different traditions, cultures and perspectives. Until recently most schools in the UK isolated themselves from or were isolated by their communities to enable them to educate the children without interruption or distraction from outside. We are, moreover, great respecters of other people's integrity, especially their professional integrity, and the notion that teachers taught and community workers worked, each in their respective areas or territories, with the boundaries carefully demarcated, surprised no-one. Professional associations and unions institutionalized the practice, and boundaries have become deeply respected, and rarely questioned.

In schools complications have arisen due to the pedagogic belief in the value of the community outside the school as an environment for learning if the process of education is to bridge childhood and adult life meaningfully and realistically. It has also heralded an era of open access schools, underpinning principles of the school as an integral part of the wider community. Experiments range from village colleges, newer purpose-built schools without recognizable lines of demarcation between campus and neighbourhood, to old and traditional schools with new policies of open and welcoming school gates positively attracting such members of the community as parents and representatives of the statutory and voluntary agencies in new partnership roles not believed possible a generation ago. These partnerships range from Taylor Report[1] type community representation on boards of governors to temporary assistance in the classroom by parent auxiliaries. Not surprisingly the most successful partnerships occur in primary schools, particularly at the first or infant school stage, where the roles of school teacher, nursery school teacher and mother overlap and where daily communication can occur as the mother collects her child from school. It is also at this level that parent auxiliaries are most frequently encountered as they assist the teacher in such tasks as reading to the children or accompanying them on a school visit. At this stage boundaries between school and community are low, permeable or non-existent.

Impediments to School-Community Cooperation

The outside world has also entered the school, uninvited, presenting a wide range of problems arising out of the continuing effects of social, economic and technological change; problems such as confusion over norms, values and patterns of behaviour, broken homes and guaranteed unemployment. The effect has been to leave teachers somewhat bemused, exposed and vulnerable as that professional group on whom society depends to 'transmit the culture' and at the same time to protect and children from such social evils as drugs, sex and alcohol. In spite of the massive build up of school pastoral care systems, and the selective appointment of teachers whose major responsibility is the social welfare of pupils, the average teacher feels singularly ill-equipped to cope with a school response to such problems. His training will hardly have prepared him. The collective and coordinated response which is required lies beyond the school's jurisdiction across the school-community divide, where until now a satisfactory level of cooperation between school and the various community agencies has not emerged to achieve the necessary network of care and education for children, particularly those at risk.[2]

In the field of health education the Schools Council Health Education Projects are as welcome to the teachers in schools as the arrival of the United States Cavalry at a beleaguered outpost. But when the dust settles, the truth remains that a new self-help and house-ordering philosophy and methodology, while a great improvement, are not enough to re-equip the garrison. Much of the knowledge and expertise needed to produce materials and design new programmes of health education lies outside the range of professional training of teachers, lodged in the minds and practices of other agencies, statutory and voluntary, 'out there' in the community. The members of such agencies range from hospital physicians and dieticians to voluntary playgroup leaders, all with their respective fields of expert knowledge. One has only to be reminded of the range of school health education curricular topics: personal health and body management, food selection, individual growth and development, social relationships, parenthood, community and environmental health, safety and first aid, etc., to realize the interdependence of school and community knowledge and expertise. However, much of what lies outside the school is not easily accessible to the teacher.

Few teachers and members of other agencies and support services fail to realize the need for a working partnership and a clearer coordination of health education policies and activities. The problem lies in the differences in experience, learning and training. These differences must be resolved before a meaningful dialogue and active cooperation can develop.

Differing Perceptions of School Health Education and Associated Roles and Tasks

Unlike the school situation where teachers, however diverse in their beliefs and methodology, are teachers, working together (albeit in their separate classrooms!) under one roof, under one headteacher, who once convinced will support the principle of the school health education coordinator, the scene outside is very different. It is much less coordinated or even open to coordination. Who would have the courage to attempt or the skill to achieve a coordination of statutory and voluntary fieldworkers, of different traditions and disciplines? Cooperation with schools is largely uncoordinated; external agencies where they do contribute to school health education programmes are usually invited to do so on a piecemeal basis. There seems to be little evidence of external agencies being involved in joint planning with schools and, therefore, little opportunity of extending possible areas of common understanding.[3]

Three interlinked problems of the internal/external view of school health education must be resolved before cooperation at a significant level can occur.

Problem 1.   What Perceptions Are There of School Health Education?

Firstly, there is the problem of the range of perceptions surrounding 'health' and 'education'. This manifests itself in confusions such as that between health care and health education. Overall, however, there is the larger and more general problem of the nature and purpose of school health education. On this, the range of external perceptions far exceeds that encountered among members of an average school staff, which in turn may be far from united.

Schools and other institutions, can be distinguished by the values they represent, which have become embodied in their educational policies, declared or implicit. Basically, these fall into four categories:

Authoritarian   Centrally agreed objectives of knowledge, attitudes and skills which pupils imbibe passively

Persuasive   Centrally agreed objectives, but pupils encouraged into more active part in studying questions to which the answers are predetermined

Autonomous   No centrally agreed objectives other than pupil autonomy; pupils enjoined to examine evidence on which to base decisions which are freely arrived at

'Social action'   Devolution of policy decision-making to autonomous groups which together represent all the interested parties.

It is not difficult to appreciate that these categories rarely exist in practice as specific schools, but that to a greater or lesser extent all four categories are found in every school. Whichever is the dominant one gives the school its distinctive character which, in turn, will strongly influence the particular interpretation of health education encountered there.

At a lower level these categories exist in school subject departments and are present in combination (and possible conflict!) in those subject departments which draw on a range of other subject disciplines, as does health education. Again, the character of health education programmes will reflect the different interpretations of different subject departments. This is recognized in the workshop strategy of the Schools Council Health Education Project which at 'Stage One' requires teachers involved in health education to reflect on their work and to review it in discussion together as a first step to the next stage, that of joint planning of future work.[4] This 'reflect and review' exercise has political implications, in that if followed through to joint planning and implementation it will inevitably lead to a power shift which will ultimately locate policy decision-making among staff in the 'social action' category. However, until a consensus has emerged in school from 'Stage One' negotiations, and a base line is established on what has been agreed among the staff, then any re-negotiation with contributors external to the school will lack a clear purpose and definition.

The external view of the school's health education role, as perceived by any of the potentially supportive agencies, will cover the same four-fold range as outlined above, the perception of individual members being shaped by their own personal and professional experience, training and beliefs, as well as by such structural considerations as the physical, social and economic make-up of the catchment area. Where, however, such individuals disagree with the values or policies of the school, they will probably not venture their personal or agency view of health education when on school territory because of their respect for the teacher's professional integrity. Thus members of external agencies may be involved in school health education programmes while holding different views of the nature of the task and the goals to be achieved. The school may be quite unaware of this dichotomy.

Problem 2:   What Perceptions Are There of the Educational Role and Methods of Work?

Secondly, and more specifically, are the different internal (school) and external perceptions of the educational role and related methods of work:

1   an individual's perception of his/her educational role and methods of work as distinct from his agency's (which usually means his line manager's), and his resolution of such issues as the 'professional versus bureaucrat' inner conflict, i.e., whether he is able to achieve a higher level of independent judgment and decision-making at the expense of bureaucratic controls;

2   the teacher and the school's perceptions of the different agencies and their representatives. This is affected considerably by such factors as school policy towards its local community and the extent to which members of school staff are allocated specific responsibilities which require close cooperation with external agencies, e.g., school-based education welfare officer, school counsellor, school nurse, community liaison officer;

3   the concept of 'partnership' in the health educational role, i.e., the teacher's realization that, without the cooperation of agencies with more detailed and up-to-date health knowledge and the cooperation of the child's parents, much of his effort will be misdirected and ineffectual. How valued is the contribution of an external agency? Should the aim be to attain an 'equal partnership' across the school-community divide?

Problem 3.   Perceptions of Teaching and Possession of Appropriate Skills

Thirdly, there are internal/external perceptions of teaching and the extent to which members of external agencies feel they are equipped with the necessary knowledge and skills, e.g., their training may have been exclusively on communication methods in a one-to-one situation, or may have been confined to 'instruction' in a group situation.

Ancillary Problems

In addition, further factors inhibit school-community communication and cooperation.

1 Control. Who initiates? Who is in charge? How sensitive are they to other views? The fear of loss of professional autonomy in a cooperative venture.
2 Lack of appeal to the community, especially parents, if the rewards are intangible or too long-term.
3 Lack of commitment to a cooperative exercise by busy external agencies if it is to be largely a 'talking-shop' leading to little or no joint action or improvement.
4 The difficulty of a school locating members of various external agencies which have a rapid turn-over of staff.
5 The particular difficulties surrounding access to and maintaining communication with parents in the lower socio-economic groups.

Cross-Boundary In-Service Projects and the Joint Learning Process

Over the last ten years in-service policies of the University of Southampton Department of Education have come up against all of these problems in their attempt to involve members of external agencies alongside teachers in the professional interests of both groups. Two regional projects, 'Fit for Life?' and 'Families with Young Children', exemplify both the difficulties and possible methods of overcoming them.

'Fit for Life?' was the title of a series of health education in-service radio programmes mounted jointly with the local radio station, BBC Radio Solent, the District Health Education Centre, and educational, health, medical and social agencies in the region. The aim was to examine key topics in health education and approaches to teaching them in the secondary school. The programmes were 'intended to be of help to teachers, allied professionals in the health and social services, parents and other members of the community.' Ten interagency programme planning teams were created to decide the best method of presenting each of the topics. Technical assistance was provided by BBC staff. As the programmes aimed to be 'issue raising' as well as informative, 'listener groups' were planned, and fourteen were set up in different parts of the region. It was hoped that, overall, the radio programmes and associated discussions by interagency groups on such matters as the place of health education in the curriculum, the content of courses, methods of approach to the 'key topics' and the roles and interrelationships of the various agencies might advance joint thinking, if not joint action.

However, the attempt at formal evaluation of the broadcasts and discussions which subsequently occurred was defeated by technological progress! Instead of the programmes being followed as a series, they were recorded by the various enterprising listener groups who then evolved their own programmes of discussion independently of the order of the broadcast series, several on an entirely different time scale to suit the convenience of their members. Questionnaire returns were therefore insufficient to form an overall clear impression of listener group opinion. However, selective follow-up interviews indicated one widespread characteristic: teachers, parents and members of the different agencies who had hitherto never even met each other, much less worked together, now discovered a common purpose and benefit in the process of meeting regularly as a group to pursue health education matters. Such meetings continued for some months in different parts of the region after the radio series had ended; some may still continue.

A later project, '*Families with Young Children*',[5] organized jointly by Hampshire Area Health Authority and Hampshire County Council in association with the University of Southampton Department of Education and Department of Sociology and Social Administration, established inter-agency working groups in six centres in Hampshire, with a view to exploring the joint learning process more fully. The objectives were:

1 to provide the means for fieldworkers [members of health, social and educational agencies working in the community] to examine their role definition and level of interprofessional communication and action within their local areas;
2 to generate material from such examination for later use in inter-disciplinary training and service planning;
3 to create opportunities for learning, especially about family support systems in communities;
4 to field-test an approach to interdisciplinary in-service training.

These were pursued over a six-month period by groups which included primary school teachers, health visitors, education welfare officers, social workers, playgroup organizers and other LEA and voluntary community workers. Each group was led by one of a team of tutors drawn from the University Departments of Education, Psychology, Sociology and Social Administration, and Community Medicine. In the subsequent evaluation one finding related to the fourth objective is particularly significant in view of later developments in Basingstoke, one of the centres.

The group members, however, did find time to explore some of their professional needs and priorities, and made a case for doing so on a regular basis. Furthermore, the opportunity provided by the Project for exchanging information and opinions in a 'non-threatening' situation led to some identification and lowering of inter-agency barriers, and, more positively, for a wish to explore and promote ways of sharing certain aspects of training at initial and post-experience stages, particularly in their local areas. In view of this, there would appear to be advantages in developing an action-research model to assist inter-agency functioning in local areas. It is important to point out that although group members demonstrated a desire to render inter-agency barriers less opaque in order to further understanding and trust and, ultimately, co-operation, there was a strong residual belief that professional identities should be preserved.[6]

As in the case of 'Fit for Life', participants found themselves in close agreement over the value of the joint learning process.

The common basis to the two projects was a methodology which, incidentally, would have been recognized by Paulo Freire,[7] and which is now becoming an increasingly accepted part of adult education, continuing education and teacher and interagency in-service training. Essentially, it is based on developing the capacity of 'critical consciousness' among individuals by inviting them to address themselves in an interagency group to three sets of basic questions:

1 What are the problems? Can we define them more clearly? (Freire's stage of 'identification')
2 Why do they exist? What factors can we identify? What weighting should we allocate to the factors? (Freire's stage of 'reflection')
3 How can the situation be improved? What contribution can we make? (Freire's stage of 'action')

In one sense what the 'rogue' self-programming listener groups in the 'Fit for Life' series achieved was the stage of critical reflection; the group members engaging in dialogue together in their search for meaning among the problems which they themselves had introduced and identified. This, however, falls short of Freire's stage of 'action'.

A Possible Process Model from a Community Project Working Group

Recently an interagency group which meets monthly at a community centre in Basingstoke, a new town, has set itself the task of evaluating the town planners' achievements at community level. While the project is still at an early stage, the broad representation of teachers, social workers, health visitors, midwives, policemen, the clergy, etc. in the working group, and the level of communication achieved among them, by virtue of their understanding of each other's roles, tasks, and associated constraints would indicate an articulate and carefully coordinated appraisal of the situation. This view has been further strengthened by the involvement of establishment figures and officials at the stage of 'critical reflection', i.e., the analysis of problems, of which, understandably, school and community health education is but one.

What can be learned from the Basingstoke experience which is likely to be of value in our search for a model of school-community interaction?

As Freire implies but does not 'spell out', the central task is one of successful management. One marked feature of the Basingstoke group project, apart from the demonstrable ability and desire to collectively achieve an environmental improvement, is the strong professional image and apparent autonomy of each of the members. To them there is no conflict of loyalty between membership of a community agency and membership of a working group that may report critically on the real achievements of their community services. While many teachers and members of external agencies may never have heard of Weber's 'classical model of bureaucracy', they are, nevertheless, strongly influenced by its British counterpart — a preoccupation with organizational hierarchies and an individual's position in them, and, their historical antecedents, namely social class divisions. Most of our older organizations — schools, health departments, local government offices, etc. — are dominated by organizational hierarchies, as is industry. However, in recent years some rethinking on the part of some industries of their internal structure has led to a greater emphasis on devolution of responsibility and accountability with correspondingly less emphasis on positional authority and hierarchy. More decisions are now being made at the point where the problems are most clearly perceived. Management, therefore, has a new role of facilitating lines of communication and promoting unity where before only differentiation and disunity occurred. This, incidentally, has the inevitable effect of weakening certain boundaries. Such achievements are summarized by Drucker as:[8]

1   creating a true unity;
2   harmonizing in every decision and action the requirements of the immediate and long-term futures, i.e., integrating short- and long-term objectives.

At an operational level the members of the Basingstoke working group are moving into an action-centred phase which embodies these principles through a series of carefully negotiated and defined tasks.

1   Having identified its 'problems', it is using a problem-centred approach, i.e., what is deficient/good about the environment in which we are living in Basingstoke? Specific questions are framed about each of the support services.
2   Task objectives are clarified in consultation and by agreement with other members of the group.
3   A team of motivated individuals is created, all of whom have a specific responsibility and a contribution to make. Individuals thus see the team as a productive relationship, both for themselves and for the declared objectives.
4   'Benchmarks' are established for assessing progress and as stages for 'feeding back' to interested parties, such as line managers.

25

5 Professional expertise is developed, and through it greater self-confidence and self-esteem.

6 'Complementary' rather than conflicting perspectives on roles and tasks are established.

7 There is a commitment to continual reappraisal and renewal of the way of working. 'No organisation or structure has a divine right to a continued existence.'

The parallels with possible initiatives in the health education field are fairly obvious. Given time, however, and by engaging patiently and methodically step by step in a Basingstoke-type collaboration exercise, school and community agencies will together marshall the resources needed for a coherent and viable school health education programme. In Basingstoke it is hoped to set up a series of interagency workshops in health education which will include the health education teams of specific schools. The purpose will be to explore together the health education task, respective roles and methods of work. This small project, which will be funded by a national organization, will include a monitoring and evaluation of the workshops. The results could provide more detailed guidance for us in our search for 'the model'.

Who Coordinates the Community Response?

The final question then becomes to whom or where does one look to fulfil the role of coordinator or leader of the health education working group. In the UK it will probably be resolved in accordance with the extent to which the various boundaries that exist between school and community and between the various agencies themselves have been rendered less opaque, lowered or removed.

If the school-community boundary is ill-defined and the school health education coordinator enjoys the confidence and support of parents and community agencies, then his or her location in the school will be instrumental to achieving a closely integrated programme involving the outsiders in consultation, planning, providing resources, teaching, etc. If, on the other hand, boundaries are still clearly defined between agencies, and, particularly, around the school, the scope is more limited, and piecemeal initiatives may have to suffice at whatever point communication, trust and opportunities for cooperative activities present themselves across the boundaries.

The wide variety of interpretations possible at local level depends upon the priorities, policies and strategies of area and district health authorities and of local education authorities. Those health authorities which regard the education of the next generation as a high priority may have appointed a health education officer[9] with a school liaison function as one of his duties or designated a community physician to coordinate the health and social agencies' response to school health education needs. Similarly, local education authorities which have anticipated the problem of their schools attempting to relate to various external agencies may have appointed an adviser specifically for school health education and an advisory committee charged with promoting the right connections and generally coordinating the work and monitoring progress.

Certain recent developments nationally in the UK, however, may make this interactive process less of a chance occurrence than it may at first appear.

1   The increasing involvement of parents in school matters in an advisory and consultative capacity, both informally through parent-teacher associations and formally through boards of governors, many of which now have parent representatives.

2   About 400 health education officers are now in post in the majority of districts (local communities) throughout England and Wales. While their background and training for the work may be diverse and sometimes unequal to the task, they are, nevertheless, potentially the community's answer to the school-based coordinator, in that they are consultants who can be called in to advise schools, channels of communication to specialized services, and 'catalysts' whose function is to stimulate thought and action on health matters. As they are still a comparatively recent feature of community health education, questions of 'status', their political role and resources at their command await a clearer resolution.

3   The devolution of more powers to local (district) level as the National Health Service undergoes its next round of reorganization. It is possible that the presence of a stronger NHS at local level, more sensitive to local needs and priorities and in time a more effective community partner in school health education, may help to enhance the district health education officer's school liaison role and, in so doing, the quality of school health education.

In a system open to as many local interpretations of 'who coordinates the community response to school health education', perhaps the only realistic solution is to build on what we have. This would mean that rather than concern ourselves with 'who coordinates?' we should be asking 'what are the tasks, roles and skills required of a co-ordinator?' While it would be invaluable to have a nationally inspired and supported pilot enquiry in order to establish guidelines, the inescapable conclusion is that ultimately only at local level in every part of the country will that particular profile emerge, after negotiation, which will meet the complex needs of that particular school-community interface. How one fits the profile to the person or the person to the profile is the responsibility of those who decide policies, strategies and methods.

George Campbell (UK)

Notes

1 Taylor Report (1977) *A New Partnership for Our Schools*, London, HMSO.
2 Merrison Report (1979) Royal Commission on the National Health Service, London, HMSO.
3 *Ibid.*
4 Schools Council Health Education 13–18 Project (1978) *Co-ordinator's Manual*, London, Schools Council.
5 POULTON, G. and CAMPBELL, G. (Eds) (1979) *Families with Young Children — A Hampshire-Based Study Project*, Hampshire Area Health Authority and Hampshire County Council in association with the University of Southampton Department of Education and Department of Sociology and Social Administration.
6 *Ibid.*, p. 35.
7 P. FREIRE (1969) *Pedagogy of the Oppressed* New York, Herder and Herder.
8 P.F. DRUCKER (1954) *The Practice of Management*, New York, Harper Bros.
9 Cohen Report (1964) *Health Education — A Report of a Joint Committee of the Central and Scottish Health Service Councils*, HMSO.

Part 2. Policies, Strategies and Methods of Achieving Understanding and Cooperation

Introduction

Lloyd J. Kolbe and Donald C. Iverson jointly present a chapter; 'Integrating School and Community Efforts to Promote Health: Strategies, Policies and Methods'. They first demonstrate the need for a strategic integration of school and community health promotion efforts (a) to attain community *input* for the design of school health education programmes, (b) to acquire community support for the *implementation* and maintenance of health education programmes in schools, and (c) to achieve health related behavioural *impacts*. They then consider policies and methods which could be employed to achieve the above, and identify six groupings of community organizations important in the school-community collaborative process: official agencies; voluntary agencies; professional associations; sponsored agencies; civic, religious or social organizations; consumer services. Their final section is a detailed study of policies and methods which establishes, among other points, the means of involving the child's family in the health education partnership and process.

Two associated chapters, 'Teenagers and Beginning Smoking' by Herbert D. Thier, and 'Youth and Decision-making Dilemmas: New Approaches to Smoking Uptake and Prevention' by Martin V. Covington, provide appropriate exemplars from their research. Thier's chapter proposes an interventionist strategy, currently being researched, designed to prevent or postpone regular smoking. The research project's approach to intervention highlights (1) intervention experiences based on real life dilemmas which emphasize confronting the subject with choices to encourage a self-analysis of decision-making processes; (2) interventions which focus on problems of power, affiliation and social interaction concerns of adolescents rather than merely on the act of smoking. The project's intervention materials will be sensitive to issues concerning: (1) the individual's self-concept and perceptions of social inadequacy; (2) culture-specific interpersonal behavioural patterns of adolescents; and (3) the effects of cigarette smoking upon perceptions of role.

Covington's chapter concerns itself with decision-making dilemmas and their resolution which are experienced by young people, particularly in respect of smoking. From a study of the dynamics of smoking, theories are emerging which may signpost interventionist strategies. The research and development project in which he is engaged aims to help individuals to manipulate their own legitimate intentions, balancing one against another in such a manner that the individual chooses a course of action perceived as a 'best possible solution', thus providing a more permanent basis for dealing with a whole range of health-risk issues.

A discussion of the points raised in these chapters is set out in the Appendix pp. 213–7.

Integrating School and Community Efforts to Promote Health: Strategies, Policies and Methods

Lloyd J. Kolbe and Donald C. Iverson

The Need for Strategic Integration of School and Community Health Promotion Efforts

In the Carnegie Study of the Education of Educators, Charles Silberman wrote:

> If our concern is with education . . . we cannot restrict our attention to the schools, for education is not synonymous with schooling. Children — and adults — learn outside school as well as — perhaps more than — in school. To say this is not to denigrate the importance of the school; it is to give proper weight to all the other educating forces in American society; the family and the community; student peer groups; television and the mass media; the armed forces; corporate training programs; libraries, museums, churches, · boy scout troops, 4-H clubs. . . .[1]

The Secretary of the US Department of Education, Terrel Bell, recognized that children's abilities are indeed the products of such a multifarious educational environment when (in 1975) he suggested to the American Association of School Administrators that, 'The key to dramatic progress in American education is to gain a rededication to learning in the home ... schools cannot educate the youth of America without the solid support and backing of the families, the homes, and the communities from which these children come.'[2]

These premises seem especially applicable and particularly important to education about health for three strategic and related reasons. First, school health education programs are expected to address the unique health needs and interests of the community that the school serves. Thus, appropriate student, parent, and community *input* is required to plan school health education programs. Second, the *implementation* and maintenance of health education programs in schools require the active support and involvement of the community. Third, in addition to improving understanding about health, health education holds the potential to increase the abilities of individuals to make decisions and engage in behaviors that would enhance their health. To realize these potential *impacts*, however, relevant school health education activities need to be planned and implemented in concert with distinct community health promotion efforts in order to address the multiple factors in the student's environment that influence targeted health related behaviors. Therefore, school and community health promotion efforts need to be strategically integrated: (a) to attain community *input* for the design of school health education programs, (b) to acquire community support for the *implementation* and maintenance of health education programs in schools, and (c) to achieve health related behavioral *impacts*.

Generic and Strategic Policies That Entail School and Community Collaboration

Some of the policies[3] that call for school and community collaboration are generic in the sense that they do not specify whether such collaboration is to secure input for school health education programs, to foster support for program implementation and maintenance, or to ensure that factors which influence targeted behaviors are addressed coordinately within the school and within the community. For instance, a *generic* policy simply may suggest that 'school and community agencies should work together to foster the health of children and youth.' Other policies are strategic in that they specify that the purpose of collaboration is to achieve one or some combination of the three objectives identified above. For instance, a *strategic* policy might require that 'the school health education program should be planned with appropriate input from students, parents, and relevant health agencies in the community.'

Although the authors of this report are most familiar with policies in the United States, both generic and strategic polices are internationally evident. For example, in the mid-1960s, the International Bureau of Education and the United Nations Educational, Scientific and Cultural Organization (UNESCO) conducted a comparison of health education programs in the primary schools of ninety-four countries.[4] Officials from sixty-four of these nations identified 'extra-scholastic institutions dealing with health education' in their nation, and briefly described the nature of such school and community collaboration. Also in the mid-1960s, with assistance provided by officials in ninety-four countries, the World Health Organization (WHO) and UNESCO jointly sponsored the development of a sourcebook, *Planning for Health Education in Schools*.[5] The sourcebook was designed to be used internationally as an agenda for agencies planning health education programs in schools and in teacher preparation institutions. Importantly, programmatic procedures for agencies to consider are described not only in the context of the three components of the school health program (i.e., school health instruction, services, and environment), but also in the fourth context of 'school, home, and community relationships'. Other published policies that call for the integration of school and community efforts have been prepared by the World Health Organization,[6] the WHO Regional Office for South-East Asia,[7] the WHO Regional Office for Europe,[8] the Ministry of Health for the Government of India,[9] the Joint Commission on Health and Education in the USSR,[10] the Republic of the Philippines,[11] and the Canadian Education Association.[12]

In the United States school and community collaboration to promote health was called for (in 1924) in the first Report of the Joint Committee on Health Problems in Education of the National Education Association and the American Medical Association,[13] in subsequent revisions of that Report,[14] and in six editions of *Suggested School Health Policies* issued by the Joint Committee (the latest of which[15] was published in 1966). The integration of school and community health education activities in the United States also has been called for by the National Parents and Teachers Association (PTA),[16] the Interagency Conference on School Health Education;[17] the American Alliance for Health, Physical Education, and Recreation,[18] the American School Health Association;[19] the American Public Health Association;[20] the American Academy of Pediatrics;[21] the

Table 1. Common Community Organizations which could Collaborate with Schools to Promote Health

Official agencies	Voluntary agencies	Professional Associations
health department	red cross	coalition of health educators
fire department	heart association	medical society
sanitation department	diabetes foundation	dental society
water department	community health council	nursing association
	visiting nurse association	social workers' association
	planned parenthood	
Sponsored agencies	Civic, religious, or social organizations	Consumer services
life insurance	churches	pharmacies
health insurance	4-H club	hospitals
dairy council	Boy Scouts/Girl Scouts	doctors
cereal institute	YWCA/YMCA	dentists
	Kiwanis, Optimists, Lions Club, etc.	groceries
	League of Women Voters	newspapers, radio, TV
	Chamber of Commerce	

Source: Adapted from Rash, J. and Pigg, M. (1979) *The Health Education Curriculum*, New York, John Wiley, p. 48.

Education Commission of the States;[22] and the National Committee on Guidelines for Comprehensive School Health Education Programs.[23]

All the international and national policies identified can be categorized as generic or strategic. In addition, strategic policies and associated methods to integrate school and community health promotion activities further can be classified according to whether they are designed to attain community input, to acquire support for program implementation, or to achieve health related behavioral impacts. As depicted in Table 1, there are at least six types of organization (common to most communities) that could collaborate strategically with schools to promote health. These include: (1) official agencies; (2) voluntary agencies (including foundations); (3) professional associations; (4) sponsored agencies; (5) civic, religious, or social organizations; and (6) consumer services.

Management Procedures to Facilitate Strategic Integration

To effectively facilitate the strategic integration of efforts by such numerous and diverse agencies, two management procedures consistently have been called for by various international and national policies. One is to employ a trained professional (frequently referred to as a *school health coordinator*) to integrate school and community activities. (The role and functions of a school health coordinator have been described by numerous authors.[24]) The other procedure frequently entailed by various policies is the establishment of an *advisory committee*, comprising relevant school and community representatives, to provide for the integration of school and community health promotion efforts.[25] Since its function is different, such a committee should be distinguished both from the school health council (composed mainly of various school personnel concerned with health aspects of a given school system), and from the community health council (composed of various representatives concerned with health aspects of a given community). Often without the appropriate mandate, representatives, or resources, however, the school or community health council will be assigned the task of integrating school and community health promotion efforts as part of its broader responsibilities.

Although infrequently cited within policy documents, two other management procedures have been proposed to facilitate integration of school and community efforts. First, an existing or newly-created *agency* may be designated to provide for the integration of school and community health promotion efforts. For some communities a regional health education center may assume this responsibility;[26] in others a private community health clinic,[27] or the local health department may undertake the assignment.

Second, a *system* may be devised and established to provide a broad operational mechanism by which numerous relevant agencies formally are assigned discrete responsibilities and tasks required for the effective integration of school and community health promotion activities. Thus, rather than one individual, one agency, or an advisory committee assuming responsibility for integration, various relevant agencies are obliged (as part of their organizational requirements) to provide for such integration. To realize synergistic results, Simonds has proposed the development of a system that would strategically integrate the delivery of health education in at least five key settings; educational institutions (public and private schools, colleges and universities); health organizations (voluntary health agencies, health departments and other official agencies); health care facilities (hospitals, HMOs, clinics, ambulatory care centers); media organizations (television, radio, newspaper); and employment settings (business and industry).[28]

> To be comprehensive from the standpoint of practice, health education must first and foremost be planned and carried out using a systems view of human behavior — one which recognizes that there are almost always multiple causes of behavior and multiple interventions required to change it. In this sense, health education cannot be planned in isolation from other change strategies and intervention approaches.... To be comprehensive from the standpoint of organizational arrangements, health education must be planned and carried out among the major providers in society that have established responsibilities for the health and education of the populace. It is the organizational dimensions of a comprehensive health education delivery system ... [that] provide the greatest potential for new legislation, institutional arrangements and the allocation of resources.[29]

Approximating such a system, the Florida Department of Education has developed and implemented a 'Comprehensive Health Education Management Model': 1 to utilize official, professional, and voluntary health and educational resources for improvement of health education, and 2 to promote health education as an integral component of the state's health and education activities.[30]

The employment of an individual, an agency, an advisory committee, or a system to integrate school and community efforts does not imply mutually exclusive operations. In fact, effective integration most likely would result from some combination of these four management procedures to attain community input, acquire support for program implementation, and achieve health related behavioral impacts.

Policies and Methods to Attain Community Input for School Health Education Programs

Typical of strategic policies calling for school and community collaboration to plan health education programs, the WHO Regional Office for South-East Asia recommended that:

> The health education curriculum in schools should be developed in terms of pupils' needs and interests, related to personal and community health problems, and should be co-operatively planned. Since local circumstances differ, it is necessary to allow for flexibility in the curriculum to take care of local needs.[31]

Involving students, parents, school officials, and relevant community members and agencies in planning school health education programs can be instrumental: (1) to ascertaining the health needs of the community; (2) to establishing an accepted rationale for the program; (3) to ensuring that those involved in the planning understand their respective roles and responsibilities in the contemplated program; and (4) to ensuring broad support for program implementation and maintenance.

As part of the planning process, health and social service agencies can contribute to the development of an epidemiological profile (or characteristics[32]) of the community. Using the epidemiological data provided, those participating in program planning can conduct various informal and formal needs assessment activities to ascertain the interests, perceived needs, and programmatic concerns of the community.[33] Community organizations then can plan specific means by which they respectively might collaborate with schools to coordinately address designated interests, needs, and concerns. Importantly, broad community participation in program planning can generate broad commitment to the program, and widespread support for its implementation and maintenance. In addition, schools thus can serve an integral function within the comprehensive community health planning process.[34]

Policies and Methods to Acquire Community Support for Program Implementation and Maintenance

Students, parents, school personnel and relevant community members and agencies can be instrumental (1) in organizing support for the adoption, improvement, or maintenance of health education programs in schools; and (2) in securing and providing in-kind (i.e., human), financial, and material resources for program adoption, improvement or maintenance. Illustrative of strategic policies that entail community support for program implementation and maintenance, participants of the Interagency Conference on School Health Education resolved that:

> Official, voluntary, and professional health and education organizations should work together to promote improved school health

education in whatever ways they can. They should work together locally, state wide, and nationally.[35]

Conference participants also resolved that:

> 'teacher preparation in health education should be improved. Voluntary agencies in particular should do what they can to promote scholarships and funds for ·... in-service education.[36]

In the US each state is independently responsible for authorizing curriculum requirements, as well as for appropriating resources to attain such requirements. However, the capacity for state legislation actually to increase or improve health education within local schools remains somewhat dubious.[37] Rather, the existence and quality of health education programs in schools seem more a function of local community support and organization for such programs.

Methods for promoting school health education at the local level have been described by various authors.[38] Importantly, in 1975 the National PTA was funded by the US Bureau of Health Education (over a five-year period) to enable the PTAs of thirteen states to independently formulate and execute various activities designed to initiate or improve health education in local schools of their state. An analysis of methods applied and experiences gained suggested that, 'while the approaches differed significantly, their success has been facilitated by one common factor: a broad community support system.'[39] Synthesizing the understandings achieved within the various states, a manual subsequently was published to delineate how communities might organize to initiate, improve, or maintain health education programs in schools.[40]

Community members and agencies also can provide in-kind, financial, and material resources for school health education programs. For example (as recommended by the American Association for Health, Physical Education, and Recreation in 1955), relevant community members and agencies can make the latest health information available to school personnel; provide teaching aids; help in the preparation of resource units; help with special short-term projects; help with in-service education of teachers; participate in the recruitment and pre-service education of school health personnel; provide the means for demonstrations and studies; enrich the curriculum; interpret the school health program and unmet needs to the community; and help in interpretation to parents.[41]

Some school systems provide in-service experiences for relevant teachers to acquaint them with community health concerns, resources, and personnel; and to concomitantly acquaint community personnel with school health concerns, resources, and personnel.[42] Other school systems have prepared charts (which are keyed to the system's health education curricula) that identify community agencies which can provide assistance with specific health topics, and that also describe the type of services which the agency can provide (e.g., teaching packets, speakers, in-service and consulting, audiovisual materials, information on health careers, direct services to students, volunteers for classroom activities, resource identification).[43] Still other systems have enabled students to compile and update such a directory as part of their health education program.[44]

The use of volunteers in the classroom can be helpful in extending the number of people available to assist the teacher. Parents, retired persons, college students, and those with special health expertise can contribute meaningfully to the school health program.[45]

In turn, schools can provide important resources for the implementation of community health activities. As suggested by the Canadian Education Association, schools can provide facilities (e.g., classrooms, physical education facilities, home economics laboratories) as well as personnel (e.g., health educators, nurses, physical educators, home economists) for community health education efforts.[46]

Policies and Methods to Achieve Health Related Behavioral Impacts

In addition to improving understanding about health, health education holds the potential to increase the abilities of individuals to make decisions and engage in behaviors that would enhance their health. To realize this potential, however, relevant school health *education* activities need to be planned and implemented in concert with distinct school and community health *promotion* efforts in order to address the various factors in the students' environment that influence targeted health related behaviors.[47] Thus, in order to enjoy health as well as the educational outcomes, distinct school and community efforts must be integrated synergistically. As described by Green:

> The potential of health education is limited only by its inadequate integration with other sources of influence on health — economic, social, legal, and environmental....
>
> The proper understanding and use of health education, then, is in the context of the several determinants of behavior and health. Isolating it in the classroom or the clinic without regard for the family, the peers, the economics and the genetics or environments that will reinforce, enable, and predispose the intended behavioral and health outcomes can only lead to a temporary or partial achievement of these outcomes. Teachers and clinicians must look beyond their immediate contacts with students and patients. They must not allow their health education to be shut in or shut out from the broader community and family networks in which health and behavior develops and deteriorates.[48]

As an example of a strategic policy to achieve health related behavioral impacts, a report on Guidelines for Comprehensive School Health Education Programs maintains that:

> The paramount goal of comprehensive school health education is to enhance the competencies of individuals to make decisions regarding their personal and family health, and the health of the populations of which they are part. School health education programs can effectively contribute to enhancing health behaviors and the health status of the population only according to the extent to which they function in concert with distinct school and community health promotion activities that have been designed specifically to enable and reinforce targeted health behaviors.[49]

Health related behaviors of children and youth that are addressed by school health education programs also are influenced by: (1) students' families; (2) peers; (3) media; and (4) relevant community services. Methods to achieve health related behavioral impacts can be differentiated according to which of these four influences the method is designed to address.

Substantial evidence indicates that the involvement of the child's family is critical to the success of any intervention program.[50] The involvement of parents as partners in the educational enterprise can provide an ongoing system to enable and reinforce the effects of the program while it is in operation, and help sustain the effects after the program ends.[51] Schools systematically can stimulate and assist parents to enable and reinforce targeted health behaviors by simultaneously providing relevant health education classes and materials for parents;[52] by assigning 'home health projects' that require the participation of the student and his family;[53] by preparing a periodic student health report for the student and his or her family (for analysis and possible parent follow-up);[54] and by regular teacher and parent visits.[55]

Health related behaviors targeted in school health programs can be reinforced through community youth activities.[56] School-based learning can be complemented by coordinated community experiences among peer groups at community recreation facilities and in such organizations as 4-H Clubs, Girl Scouts and Boy Scouts, Junior Red Cross, church youth groups, YWCA and YMCA.

The local media in the community also can serve to reinforce targeted health related behaviors. Newspaper articles, printed flyers and brochures, mass mailings, popular radio personalities, and television announcements or programs can augment school health education programs.

Finally, students, parents, school personnel, and community health officials can work cooperatively toward ensuring that relevant health services are not only available to students, but are also familiar, accessible, and acceptable. For example, we might expect school education about venereal disease to be more effective in eliciting treatment-seeking behavior if diagnostic and treatment services were arranged to be available in the community; if students were informed about the services; if the services were arranged to be provided at an accessible time, location, and cost; and if the services were arranged to be rendered confidentially and with respect for the student's dignity.

Summary and Conclusions

The purposeful integration of school and community efforts may be *the* critical element in a formula to promote the health of school-aged children and youth. Obviously there are numerous strategies, policies, and methods to functionally integrate school and community activities. As noted by the Director of the US Office of Maternal and Child Health, 'what is required, then, are not new policies in school health, but a reaffirmation and implementation of policies that have been with us for many years.'[57]

Notes

1 SILBERMAN, C. (1976) 'The Carnegie Study of the Education of Educators: Preliminary statement of intent', in CREMIN, L. *Public Education*, New York, Basic Books, pp. 11–12.
2 BELL, T. (1975) *American Association of School Administrators Convention Reports*, Arlington, V., American Association of School Administrators.
3 For the purposes of this paper a policy is considered to be a written principle, plan, or course of action pursued by an organization.
4 International Bureau of Education and United Nations Educational, Scientific and Cultural Organization (1967) *Health Education in Primary Schools*, Geneva, International Bureau of Education.
5 TURNER, C. (1966) 'WHO and UNESCO promote planning for health education in schools and institutions for the preparation of teachers', *Journal of School Health*, 36, 10, pp. 473–80; United Nations Educational, Scientific and Cultural Organization and World Health Organization (1966) *Planning for Health Education in Schools*, Paris, UNESCO.
6 World Health Organization (1974) *Health Education: A Programme Review*, Geneva, WHO, pp. 17–18.
7 World Health Organization Regional Office for South East Asia (1956) *School Health Education in South East Asia*, New Delhi, Patiala House, pp. 10–12.
8 World Health Organization Regional Office for Europe (1977) *Evaluation of School Health Programmes*, Copenhagen, World Health Organization Regional Office for Europe, pp. 21–2.
9 Ministry of Health of the Government of India (1965) *Report of the School Health Committee*, New Delhi, Ministry of Health of the Government of India, pp. 89–90.
10 World Health Organization (1963) *Health Education in the USSR*, Geneva, WHO pp. 50–1.
11 Republic of the Philippines Department of Education and Department of Health (1964) *A Cooperative and Coordinated School Health Program of the Department of Education and the Department of Health*, Manila, Joint Circular No. 1s 1964, 17 August.

12 Canadian Education Association (1978) *Canadian Approaches to School Health Education and Services*, Toronto, Canadian Education Association, pp. 55–7.
13 Joint Committee on Health Problems in Education of the National Education Association and the American Medical Association (1924) *Health Education: A Program for Public Schools and Teacher Training Institutions*, n.p., pp. 78–9.
14 Joint Committee on Health Problems in Education of the National Education Association and the American Medical Association (1941) *Health Education: A Guide for Teachers in Elementary and Secondary Schools and Institutions for Teacher Education*, Washington, D.C., National Education Association, pp. 171–6.
15 Joint Committee on Health Problems in Education of the National Education Association and the American Medical Association (1966) *Suggested School Health Policies*, Chicago, Ill., American Medical Association, pp. ix–xii.
16 National Education Association and American Medical Association Joint Committee on Health Problems in Education (1937) *Home and School Cooperation for the Health of the School Child* (report prepared in cooperation with the National Congress of Parents and Teachers), Washington, D.C., National Education Association.
17 Interagency Conference on School Health Education (1958) *Improving School Health through Interagency Cooperation*, n.p.
18 American Alliance for Health, Physical Education, and Recreation (1962) *Teamwork in School Health* (A Report on the National Conference on Coordination of the School Health Program), Reston, Va., American Alliance for Health, Physical Education, and Recreation; American Alliance for Health, Physical Education, and Recreation (1970) 'A unified approach to health teaching', *School Health Review*, 1, 3, p. 12.
19 American School Health Association (1975) *Compendium of Resolutions, Governing Council Actions, and Position Papers of the American School Health Association*, Kent, Ohio, American School Health Association, p. Community Health-1.
20 American Public Health Association (1975) 'Education for health in the school community setting', *American Journal of Public Health*, 65, 2, p. 201.
21 American Academy of Pediatrics Committee on School Health (1978) 'Health education', *Pediatrics*, 62, 1, p. 117.
22 Education Commission of the States (1981) *Recommendations for School Health Education: A Handbook for State Policy Makers*, Denver, Colo., Education Commission of the States, pp. 4–5.
23 National Committee on Guidelines for Comprehensive School Health Education Programs (1981) *Guidelines for Comprehensive School Health Education Programs (Draft)*. San Francisco, Calif., National Center for Health Education.
24 CURTIS, J. and PAPENFUSS, R. (1980) *Health Instruction: A Task Approach*, Minneapolis, Minn., Burgess, pp. 40–4; ANDERSON, C.L. and CRESWELL, W.H. (1980) *School Health Practice*, St Louis, Mo., Mosby, pp. 117–18; BRUESS, C.E. and GAY, J.E. (1978) *Implementing Comprehensive School Health*, Riverside, N.J. Macmillan; RASH, J. and PIGG, R. (1979) *The Health Education Curriculum*, New York, John Wiley, pp. 43–5; KIME, R., SCHLAADT, R. and TRITSCH, L. (1977) *Health Instruction: An Action Approach*, Englewood N.J., Prentice-Hall p. 346; BEDWORTH, D. and BEDWORTH, A. (1978) *Health Education: A Process for Human Effectiveness*, Scranton, Pa., Harper and Row, pp. 225–9; NEMIR, A. and SCHALLER, W. (1975) *The School Health Program*, Philadelphia, Pa., Saunders, pp. 362–3; MAYSHARK, C., SHAW, D. and BEST, W. (1977) *Administration of School Health Programs*, St Louis, Mo., Mosby, pp. 92–113; BRADLEY, C. (1978) Role and function of a school health education coordinator' (mimeo), Madison, Wisc., Wisconsin Department of Public Instruction.
25 LIGHTNER, M. (1976) The health education coordinating council', *Health Education*, 7, 6, pp. 25–6.
26 DORAN, P., STRAND, G. and MEADER, J. (1974) 'A state health education resource center', *School Health Review*, 5, 4, 9–13; SORENSEN, A. and SINACORE, J. (1979) 'Developing a regional health education program', *Health Values*, 3, 2, 79–84;

HEALTH EDUCATION CENTER (1980) *Guidelines for Planning and Implementing School Health Education Programs*, Pittsburgh, Pa., Health Education Center.

27 REESE, D. (1979) 'Adolescent health: A systems approach', (mimeo), Nampa, Idaho, Community Health Clinics.

28 SIMONDS, S. (1974) 'Considerations for the design of a comprehensive health education delivery system, *Papers on Theoretical Issues in Health Education: Dorothy Nyswander International Symposium*, Berkeley, Calif, p. 175.

29 SIMONDS, S. (1977) 'Health education today: Issues and challenges', *Journal of School Health*, 47, 10, p. 587.

30 US Bureau of Health Education (1980) *Comprehensive Health Education Management Model*, Atlanta, Ga., US Bureau of Health Education.

31 World Health Organization Regional Office for South East Asia (1956) *op. cit.*, p. 10.

32 During planning there should be a differentiation between the health related *characteristics* of a community (e.g., morbidity patterns), and the *needs* of a community. A need might be thought of as a perceived discrepancy between an existing state and a preferred state. Thus, the identification of needs and the ranking of need priorities require decisions based on personal or group values.

33 NEWMAN, I. and MAYSHARK, C. (1973) 'Community health problems and the schools' unrecognized mandate', *Journal of School Health*, 43, 9, pp. 562–5; GILMORE, G. (1977) 'Needs assessment processes for community health education', *International Journal of Health Education*, 20, 3, 164–73; THYGERSON, A. (1977) 'Task analysis: Determining what should be taught', *Health Education*, 8, 2, pp. 8–9; KUNSTEL, F. (1978) Assessing community needs: Implications for curriculum and staff development in health education', *Journal of School Health*, 48, 4, pp. 220–4.

34 SAYLOR, L. (1969) California's schools: An untapped resource in comprehensive health planning', *Journal of School Health*, 39, 7, pp. 487–92.

35 Interagency Conference on School Health Education (1958) *op. cit.*, p. 23.

36 *Ibid.*

37 MILLER, D. (1972) 'Legislative action, health education, and curriculum change', *Journal of School Health*, 42, 9, pp. 513–15; MEEDS, L. (1973) 'Legislation as a precipitator of educational development', *School Health Review*, 4, 5, pp. 21–5; STEIN, B. (1973) Legislative action for school health', *School Health Review*, pp. 26–9; CONLEY, J. and JACKSON, C. (1978) 'Is a mandated comprehensive health education program a guarantee of successful health education?' *Journal of School Health*, 48, 6, pp. 337–40; NEWMAN, I. and WILSON, R. (1980) 'Political action and the value of health education — a case study of community attitudes and actions in a legislative hearing', *Health Values*, 4, 3, pp. 124–9.

38 GRACE, H. (Ed.) (1978) *Comprehensive Health Education in New Mexico Public Schools: A Community Action Manual*, Albuquerque, New Mexico, New Mexico PTA; CURTIS and PAPENFUSS (1980) *op. cit.*, pp. 84–96; AMA Medicine/Education Committee on School and College Health (1980) *Physician's Guide to the School Health Curriculum Process*, Chicago, Ill., American Medical Association.

39 National Parents and Teachers Association (1981) *Health Education Matters*, Atlanta, Ga., US Center for Health Promotion and Education, p. 8.

40 *Ibid.*, pp. 1–39.

41 American Association for Health, Physical Education, and Recreation (1956) 'How schools and voluntary agencies can work together to improve school health programs', *School Health*, April, pp. 118–22.

42 OSWALT, L. and JUILFS, B. (1970) 'A rolling approach to community health: The rubber neck tour', *Journal of School Health*, 40, 8, pp. 414–16; BAKER, G. and RISER, M. (1971) 'Teacher education project: Community health resources', *School Health Review*, 2, 1, pp. 33–5.

43 San Mateo County Office of Education (1980) *Synopsis of health instruction framework for California public schools coded for San Mateo County interagency services*, San Mateo,

Calif., SanMateo Office of Education.

44 SROKA, S. (1977) 'Preparing a directory of community health services', *Journal of School Health*, 47, 8, 484–6.

45 HAGER, D. (1977) 'Teachers and volunteers in the classroom', in HAGER, D. *Community Involvement for Classroom Teachers*, Charlottesville, Mid-Atlantic Center for Community Education, pp. 14–21.

46 Canadian Education Association (1978) *op. cit.*, p. 33.

47 Health *education* has been defined as any combination of learning opportunities designed to facilitate voluntary adaptations of behaviors (in individuals, groups, or communities) conducive to health. In contrast, health *promotion* has been defined to include any combination of health education *and* related organizational, political, and economic interventions designed to facilitate behavioral and environmental changes that will improve or protect health. KOLBE, L. (1981) 'What can we expect from school health education?' (mimeo) paper presented at the London University Institute of Education, March 1981, San Francisco, Calif., National Center for Health Education; GREEN, L. (1980) 'Definitions from OHP', *Focal Points*, June, p. 1.

48 GREEN, L. (1979) 'The misunderstanding and misuse of health education', *Journal of School Health*, 49, 5, p. 290.

49 KOLBE, L. (1981) 'Guidelines for comprehensive school health education programs: Background paper (draft mimeo), San Francisco, Calif., National Center for Health Education, p. 5.

50 HAGER, D. (1977) 'Rationale for teachers' involvement with community', in HAGER, D. *Community Involvement for Classroom Teachers*, Charlottesville, Va., Mid-Atlantic Center for Community Education, pp. 7–13; NADER, P. (1980) *Family Directed Health Education*, Galveston, Tex., University of Texas Medical Branch.

51 BRONFENBRENNER, V. (1974) *Is Early Intervention Effective?: A Report on Longitudinal Evaluations of Preschool Programs*, Washington, D.C., US Office of Child Development, II, p. 55.

52 HOPP, J. and IRWIN, C. (1980) 'Nutrition physical fitness education for families (mimeo), presented at the annual meeting of the American Public Health Association, October 1980, Loma Linda, Calif., Loma Linda University; Michigan Department of Education (1980) *The Health Education Family Handbook*, Lansing, Mich., Michigan Department of Education.

53 Joint Committee on Health Problems in Education of the National Education Association and the American Medical Association (1924) *op. cit.*, p. 78.

54 *Ibid.*

55 DELELLIS, A. (1977) 'Home visitations', in HAGER, D. *Community Involvement for Classroom Teachers*, Charlottesville, Va., Mid-Atlantic Center for Community Education, pp. 42–51; COLARUSSO, R. (1974) 'Parent involvement', *School Health Review*, 5, 4, pp. 23–4.

56 Joint Committee on Health Problems in Education of the National Education Association and the American Medical Association (1941) *op. cit.*, p. 228.

57 HUTCHINS, V. (1977) 'New policies in school health', *Journal of School Health*, 47, 7, p. 430.

Teenagers and Beginning Smoking

Herbert D. Thier

In this paper concepts of status and role as described in Baric's Social Intervention Model of Health Education are used to define and describe becoming a teenager in relation to the individual's early uptake of smoking behavior. Evidence from the early work of the Risk and Youth: Smoking (RAY: S) project is used to describe some of the characteristics of 'beginning smoking' and how it is quite different from the 'regular smoking' of the adult smoker. A period of trial or exploratory smoking is suggested as one of the behaviors many teenagers engage in as part of the growing up process. For example, in a recent survey of over 200 Psychology 1 students at the University of California, Berkeley, over 50 per cent reported having smoked at least one cigarette, while a small percentage are currently smokers. The value of postponing as long as possible the teenager's decision to start smoking regularly is substantiated on the basis of considerations from developmental psychology and the Social Intervention Model of Health Education, and an intervention strategy is proposed which is expected to prevent or postpone regular smoking.

Status and Role

The Social Intervention Model (SIM) of Health Education (Baric, 1979) highlights the role of the individual as a member of a social system. Health behavior is considered an aspect of everyday life and not something separate. One is not concerned with the 'problem of smoking,' but rather looks at the person as an interacting member of a social system who smokes as part of his or her individual everyday lifestyle.

A person's everyday life system is integrated into the social system of the individual's social environment. Integration is at the status-role level. As used here, status represents an ideal or 'pure case' institutionalized into society, with all the rights and duties belonging to it. It may never be found completely in a real-life situation. It is the idealization of society's expectations for the individual's occupying a particular position (Gould and Kolb). Role, on the other hand, is defined as putting into action the rights and duties entailed in a status (Linton, 1936). Role, therefore, is the way the individual interprets and acts in regard to a status of which he or she is a part.

Society expects the child to take on the status of teenager at about 12 or 13 years old. Each young person fulfils this new status by taking on his or her individual perception of the role of teenager. Whereas many other social statuses, like father or mother, are defined and described by social expectations that lead to positive roles, the status teenager is usually defined by a complex series of mixed messages which frequently lead to a role including rebelliousness and alienation on the part of the young person.

According to Baric (1979), role performance is defined by a set of social expectations, and when a role is formalized, these expectations become the norms for the role and are supported by sanctions of the society. For example, society has expectations of how a father or mother should act, and so there are accepted role performances for these statuses. This is evident by the fact that even young children can accurately play-act these roles and, conversely, the fact that behaviors, such as child abuse or neglect, are clearly proscribed by society.

Unfortunately, in the case of teenagers, the social expectation is dichotomous; mixed messages are transmitted by parents, teachers, and society in general. Parents and teachers, for example, exhort teens to stop being childish, act maturely, take responsibility, etc., while telling them what they can't do, can't try, and aren't old enough for. Society in general, as evidenced by the media, encourages the young teen to join, participate, buy, consume, while passing legal restrictions on employment, smoking, drinking, and other activities. Mixed messages include 'training bras', designer jeans, and other invitations for teens to dress as adults and look sexy, while society laments teenage promiscuity. A clearly mixed message is the offering at restaurants of non-alcoholic teen drinks that look like real liquor. These mixed messages start, for example, with the candy cigarettes available for sale to young children. Physical maturation, natural curiosity, the desire for independence and the right to be 'my own boss' contribute to the typical teen's rebellious attitudes. These same factors increase the individual's desire to be part of the world as depicted by the media.

What, therefore, are the norms of this teenage group in society? By norms I mean those which Sherif and Sherif define as the 'clustering of the modal or average perceptions, attitudes, opinions or acts by members of a social group combined with the element of social constraint' (Sherif and Sherif, 1948). For teenagers this element of social constraint is not to look or act childish. Parents, the media, and society agree on this one point, even though they agree for very different reasons. For teens, however, the only obvious and viable way not to appear childish is to look and 'act' like adults.

The easiest way to achieve this model is to take on, or at least claim, overt adult behavior, such as smoking or drinking, which is forbidden to children. Young teens especially have a great need to 'identify' with the group, even if real participation in the group is not available. Sometimes the young teen will try to achieve this identity by wearing a lot of makeup or otherwise adopting an overtly adult way of dressing.

Relating all of this to our concern with smoking prevention and the young teenager, I propose the following model for the role of the individual teen. The need to identify with the group called teenagers is very strong, since being a teenager is proof of leaving childhood. The group 'teenager', however, in some ways exists primarily in advertizing promotions, other media, and general societal descriptions of teenagers. The overall effect is to encourage individuals to do or say almost anything to be able to consider themselves part of the stereotyped group, even though in many ways the group is only a media phenomenon and does not exist. The desire for group membership explains the wildfire-like spread of fad clothing and other teen symbols among teenagers.

Again, referring to Baric (1969), there is little immediate health risk to young teenagers and, therefore, it is very difficult to postulate the classic 'at-risk' role for young teens regarding smoking or any other health hazard. Teens who are not ill perceive themselves in the 'well' role, initiating their own actions, and integrated into the social system as teenagers. The teen status, as described above, provides mixed and confusing messages. Therefore, the individual teenagers trying to fulfil their status become confused and take on role performances frequently at variance with expectations parents and others have of them.

The desire is to do something that clearly shows to oneself and to others that one is no longer a child, and the act of smoking is frequently that 'something'. Children are not allowed to smoke. Smoking is depicted in the media as adult, sexy, and cool. Cigarettes (even when sales are illegal) are easily available to teens. Smoking is considered by many teens to be one way to prove they are no longer children. They do not accept an 'at-risk' role for themselves, and telling teens that smoking is bad for their health will have little effect. What is needed is a clearer understanding of the nature of teenage smoking as the basis for the design of interventions that will bring about changes in the value and importance teenagers give to smoking as a way of proving their identity. Currently, the RAY:S project is researching the nature of teenage smoking as a basis for the development of such interventions.

Nature of Beginning Smoking

In order to understand more fully the nature and dimensions of beginning smoking, we have been using both projective and retrospective techniques for collecting evidence. Thirteen and 14-year-olds have been asked to write a story in which they describe the situation in which another individual is tempted to smoke. They can choose a boy or a girl their own age (grade 8) or approximately two years younger (grade 6). In one form of the activity, the original writer describes the situation, but does not tell whether the individual smokes or not. A peer writes the end of the story. In other forms, the writer is responsible for the whole story.

We have collected such stories from over 150 eighth graders and are pleasantly surprised by the quality of the writing, as evidenced by the length and detail of the stories and the high interest of the eighth graders in participating. The sample includes a wide variety of subjects, ranging from high socio-economic status white and oriental individuals to low socio-economic status black and chicano students. Interest in the task was high in all groups, and interesting provocative stories were obtained from all groups. The chicano background students had their choice of responding in Spanish or English, and Spanish language forms of the activity were made available.

In addition to these written stories, we have carried out over 100 interviews with young teenagers in which we have asked them to talk about their own smoking, the smoking of others, and/or to react to stories about situations (dilemmas) in which teenagers are pressured to smoke. Some of these interviews are open-ended, while others are highly structured. Preliminary review of the data from all these sources indicates that similar reasons for beginning smoking are given, whether the young teen is describing his or her own smoking behavior or projecting about the behavior of other teens. Young teens relate smoking to desires for affiliation with individuals or groups. They see smoking as a reaction to being in situations where cigarettes are available, or as a way of promoting status and acceptance and warding off rejection or insult. Rarely are the taste or pleasure of cigarettes, feelings of relaxation, or just curiosity mentioned as important reasons for beginning to smoke cigarettes.

In addition to collecting this projective and current status information about smoking from young teens, we have begun to collect retrospective data from college students and other adults. In these situations the individuals are asked in writing or in person whether they ever smoked and, if so, to describe, as well as they can remember, their first smoking experience. We are amazed by the richness and detail of the responses we obtain from most adults who have smoked. Few cannot remember this first experience, and the more typical reaction, especially in interview situations, is a smile, an 'oh yes', or 'let me tell you', followed by a very detailed story. Preliminary review of these responses indicates significant differences between the retrospective descriptions given by these adults and the current status and projective descriptions given by the young teenagers. These differences are consistent with our evolving developmental model for the uptake of smoking behavior (Covington, 1981). In spite of these differences, motives directly related to the pleasure of smoking per se are rarely cited by either group.

Review and analysis of all of this naturalistic data are continuing, as is the collection of such data from additional subjects. A number of additional questions is under exploration in order to understand more fully the nature of beginning smoking. The desire to smoke for the sake of smoking (pleasure, taste, etc.) is rare.

The RAY:S Approach to Smoking Prevention

Early evidence from our work indicates that the act of smoking for the young adolescent is typically an arbitrary, instrumental means of resolving a variety of momentary dilemmas which frequently confront the individual. We are finding these are usually conflicts related to power or affiliation. This evidence, and considerations based on the project's evolving model for the uptake of smoking behavior in adolescents (Covington, 1981), lead to our postulating a 'trial period' during which many young teenagers will engage in 'exploratory behavior' regarding smoking. Our early evidence indicates this kind of smoking tends to be random, infrequent, and provoked by external incidents. From the current reports of the young teens and the retrospective descriptions of the adults, it is clear that enjoyment, good taste, etc. are not part of these early smoking experiences. Coughing, obnoxious odors, feeling sick, and 'it was terrible' are much more typical descriptions of initial smoking experiences. We are particularly interested in these descriptions of the real effects of early smoking and intend to use them in our intervention program to contradict the vastly different messages about smoking provided to the young teen by cigarette advertizing.

Additional evidence leads us to believe that the activity of smoking cigarettes is minimally associated with an intention 'to smoke' or with any cognitively-derived decision to 'become a smoker', at least for our young teenage subjects. Even when a decision per se has been made to smoke or not to smoke in a given situation, the decision is generally based on an entirely different set of issues. The act of smoking, as stated earlier, is typically an *arbitrary, instrumental* means of resolving a power or affiliation-related dilemma which momentarily confronts the adolescent. All this reduces the probability that young teens will become physiologically or psychologically addicted to smoking during this trial period. We believe that conceptualizing smoking onset as a trial or exploratory period will reduce the pressure, direct or implied, on the teenager to identify with the role of smoker.

We plan to design intervention experiences which discourage all smoking, while accepting that many teens will try cigarettes at one time or another. Our approach to intervention will highlight: (1) intervention experiences based on real-life dilemmas which are being collected by the project in its research phase and which emphasize confronting the subject with choices to encourage a self-analysis of decision-making processes; and (2) interventions which focus on problems of power, affiliation, and social interaction concerns of adolescents rather than just on the act of smoking. RAY:S intervention materials will be sensitive to issues concerning: (1) the individual's self-concept and perceptions of personal social adequacy; (2) culture-specific interpersonal behavioral patterns of adolescents; and (3) the effects of cigarette smoking upon perceptions of role.

By emphasizing in these interventions the realities of, and reasons for, trial or exploratory smoking, we expect at least to decrease such smoking and minimize acceptance of regular smoking behaviors. Theoretical considerations from developmental psychology (Covington, 1981) and the SIM Model for Health Behavior seem to substantiate the importance of at least postponing the individual's decision to adopt the 'role' of smoker. Early adolescents do not have a realistic grasp of, or interest in, long-term, cumulative health risk and consequences. They are typically concerned with immediate, concrete pay-offs, rather than long-term potentials. The assumption is that with greater maturity, cognitively and emotionally, the individual will be more likely to reject the role of smoker. Early information from the evidence we are collecting retrospectively seems to bear out this assumption. That is, many more adults report exploring smoking than those labeling themselves as smokers now. We are engaged in further research to define more clearly and further describe the existence and characteristics of this trial period.

References

BARIC, L. (1969), 'Recognition of the "at-risk" role: A means to influence health behavior', *International Journal of Health Education*, 18, 1, pp. 2–12.

BARIC, L. (1979) 'Non-smokers, smokers, ex-smokers: Three separate problems for health education', *International Journal of Health Education*, 22, 1, pp. 2–17.

COVINGTON, M.V. (1981) 'Youth and decision-making dilemmas: New approaches to smoking uptake and prevention', paper presented at the International Seminar on School Health Education, University of Southampton, 31 March to 3 April 1981.

GOULD, J. and KOLB, W.L. (Eds) (1964) *A Dictionary of the Social Sciences*, London, Tavistock Publications, p. 692.

LINTON, R. (1936) *The Study of Man*, New York, Appelton-Century, pp. 113–14.

SHERIF, M. and SHERIF, C.W. (1948) *An Outline of Social Psychology*, New York, Harper and Bros.

Youth and Decision-Making Dilemmas: New Approaches to Smoking Uptake and Prevention

Martin V. Covington

The purpose of this paper is to describe the Risk and Youth: Smoking (RAY:S) project, Lawrence Hall of Science, University of California. The overall objective of the project is to develop effective, widely applicable educational interventions which will increase the ability of young people to make informed decisions about their behavior in situations which tempt them to smoke or to engage in other activities potentially injurious to their health. The project consists of three interlocking phases: (1) a program of basic research and theory building; (2) the practical implementation of theory and research findings in the development of educational intervention techniques; and (3) field-testing and formal evaluation of these instructional products both in schools and in informal community settings. I will concentrate my remarks on our evolving theoretical formulations regarding smoking dynamics among youth and their implications for intervention.

We take as our mandate the conclusions of Leventhal and Cleary (1980) regarding the state of research on the smoking problem, in which they suggest that more comprehensive models of risk-taking behavior are needed, particularly approaches that reflect the developmental history of smoking uptake and resistance among individuals and groups. Certainly uncoordinated and often conflicting findings abound in this field, and in many instances the facts are without sufficient theoretical grounding to guide further investigation. Even in the case of the most sophisticated instances of current research — in which the probability of smoking uptake is estimated from a host of antecedent personality and environmental variables — the primary emphasis remains at the level of *prediction* of behavior. While researchers are beginning to be able to predict the kinds of youngsters who can take up smoking, those who will not, and those who will become enmeshed in a life of harder substance abuse and addiction, we remain essentially uninformed about the specific micro-dynamics of smoking uptake. For, if the processes of smoking initiation, cessation and resistance among adolescents are best understood in terms of a moment-by-moment decision-making drama, and we believe that they are, then more and different information is needed on which to base anti-smoking programs. We must surmise which points in such a decision-making belief process are most vulnerable to intervention and where it is unlikely to yield.

Decision-Making Dilemmas

Our focus, in this first stage of work, is on the discovery of the dimensions and dynamics of the decision-making/belief process in tempting situations that place the individual and group at risk for smoking. As a starting point, we invited several hundred junior high school youngsters from a variety of ethnic backgrounds and economic levels to describe situations in which children, either themselves or others, had been tempted to smoke. The following scenario based on a pastiche of various stories is representative:

> Pat was not doing very well in Mrs Johnson's class, and there was another test next period. On the way to class Pat heard girls talking in the restroom. Pat opened the door and recognized the smell of cigarette smoke before she saw the three girls from Miss Harris' class, two years ahead of her. The girls quickly exchanged concerned and resentful glances. Then one of them said, 'Hey, want a cigarette?' The first bell rang. It was time to go. Pat paused as she considered the offer instead of going to class.

From this and many other stories, we have come to suspect that the act of smoking for children is basically an *instrumental* means of dealing with non-smoking issues that confront the adolescent on a daily basis. For example, in the present scenario, the issues include: (1) Pat's need to maintain a sense of personal competency and worth by avoiding another test failure, perhaps by not going to class; (2) Pat's need to maintain a sense of social adequacy in the face of older, more 'mature' schoolmates; and (3) the older girls' interest in Pat's smoking, thereby gaining power over her so that she will not tell. Thus, Pat's decision may be only incidentally related to smoking per se, and very much entwined in issues of power, affiliation and competency. For many children cigarettes are often, in reality, one more weapon in their arsenal of techniques for coping; far less dramatic, to be sure, than trading on one's sexuality or performing dangerous stunts on a skateboard to gain attention, but nonetheless a bargaining chip in a larger game.

Moreover, cigarettes as objects have an astounding range of uses. They are highly versatile. We asked our young informants to explain why they, or others of their acquaintance, smoked. We discerned fourteen different categories of motives or reasons, ten of which appeared in at least 5 per cent of the total responses. These reasons ranged from warding off rejection or insult to gaining power over others, to representing a means for achieving interpersonal favor. Only 5 per cent of all the responses related to the alleged enjoyment and fun of smoking, while curiosity about cigarettes accounted for just over 2 per cent of the responses.

Psychologically, smoking is part of a larger pattern of involvement of individuals and groups with substances. How different this view is from that implied by some current adolescent anti-smoking programs in which children are trained primarily to resist social group pressures to smoke. While the scenario of the uninitiated innocent standing alone against the philistines is one important reality, it is by no means the most frequent kind of scenario provided by our informants. There are other realities, too. For example, the assertive social skills taught to resist peer pressure (basically a set of argumentative retorts: e.g., 'I'd be a chicken if I smoked just to impress you') appear calculated to alienate children from the very peer groups with which they must ultimately satisfy their needs for affiliation and competency. While increasing the youth's skill in refusing a cigarette, these projects do not seem likely to help the adolescent develop more stabilized social skills or greater motivation to use such skills. Another reality is that peers are not the only significant others, and in many cases not the most influential group, regarding smoking uptake and maintenance. Family members, most strikingly mothers and older brothers, promote smoking initiation in a substantial minority of our informants.

We conclude, perhaps paradoxically, that smoking behavior should not be the primary focus of anti-smoking programs. Intervention must work within the context of naturally occurring motivations, and not against them for a short-term relief from smoking. Rather, as in the case of our chosen approach, it must provide a range of problem-solving skills for coping with larger issues of personal/social significance, yet in ways that reduce the likelihood of problem resolution in favor of smoking. Our tentative evidence suggests that non-smoking youth may more readily grasp situational issues when it comes to dealing with real-life dilemmas. Moreover, we note that our smokers seem less realistic about the consequences of various solutions, sometimes conjuring up extreme and even fanciful images of what others will do to them if they reject a proffered cigarette. This tendency is likely linked to exaggerated views of the utility of cigarettes for achieving one's goals.

What might constitute issue resolution and problem formulation in a specific instance? Let us return to Pat's dilemma. If the issue remains solely that of smoking or not smoking, as might be the case in a strict health education mode, then we must rely heavily on health facts, on will-power and on cognitive controls that are not yet well developed to motivate a non-smoking decision. However, by bringing into play other positive motives that serve the larger perceived self-interest of the child, chances for a healthful outcome will be increased. What is needed is to enhance the youngster's capacity to identify these other issues, or as our interviewees best understand it, 'find all the sources of problems in the situation.' There is also the need to practise establishing a 'danger hierarchy': in effect, determining which courses of action are worse given all the likely consequences of each. In Pat's dilemma the issues may balance out, at first, heavily in favor of staying and smoking: more powerful peers would be placated and a test of Pat's ability postponed. But if the main issue is seen as the need to deal with potential failure, then a reframing of the situation has occurred. Constructive steps can now be considered that lean away from smoking involvement, and toward the solution of a more fundamental problem. In this case, Pat might decide to seek out the teacher's help for doing better in the future.

Undoubtedly, proper health beliefs will aid in tipping the balance of factors toward a non-smoking resolution, as perhaps will improved social skills. But we believe recognition of one's own larger self-interest in achieving autonomy, competency, and affiliation is the key to reducing health-risk behaviors. In this connection, youngsters, like adults, do not like to be manipulated by others. When children recognize in Pat's dilemma the power play of the older girls to subjugate her, a rejection of the smoking alternative is all the more likely.

It is hoped that instruction in this type of problem-formulation and resolution process will convince smokers and potential smokers that they do have options; and that, indeed, while there really are dilemmas, they are rarely beyond the capabilities of individuals to resolve.

Any successful anti-smoking program must also recognize that children tend to structure their decision options differently depending on their developmental levels of interpersonal reasoning. Consider another scenario:

> Jim was having trouble making friends at his new school. Most of the kids hung out at the shopping center and smoked. Jim had tried a cigarette last year and knew he really didn't like it. One day as he was leaving a store, he spotted a group of kids from school. Jim was too young to buy cigarettes, and besides he did not have any money with him. But there were cigarettes at the nearby check-out counter and the clerk was busy with a customer. Jim thought about taking a pack, and then walking out by the kids from school with the cigarettes showing obviously from his pocket.

The situation is differently construed and the issues which children identify vary depending on developmental status. For example, among younger pre-adolescents a likely resolution to Jim's dilemma might condone stealing on the grounds that the cigarettes, being inexpensive, would not be missed anyway, and there is greater perceived advantage in avoiding loneliness and rejection. This early level of reasoning is characterized by trade-off thinking; that is, balancing risks and benefits according to a concern for immediate, concrete pay-off with a minimum of personal pain or discomfort. In contrast, older children are likely to see the 'rule breaking' of stealing as the dominant issue, and reject it as an alternative despite their level of social discomfort. Incidentally, we see once again in this latter instance that smoking in the specific case is not necessarily the issue at stake, and that decisions in favor of smoking, or against it, may be determined on grounds entirely unrelated to health matters (see Figure 1).

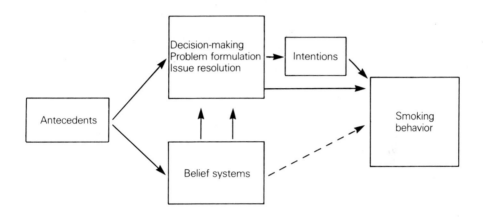

Figure 1.   A Proposed Decision-Making Model of Smoking Uptake and Resistance

Figure 1 shows a proposed model of health-risk decision-making. This is presented in a horizontal mode with the directional arrows indicating potential pathways of causation. Here we shall only trace out the most obvious relationships in this network. Smoking dilemmas, with all the decision-making, problem-formulation dynamics implied, assume a central place. Those dilemma outcomes of special interest to us are the children's reasoning in reaching various decisions, and how they themselves resolve each conflict. We assume that those projected, hypothetical decisions are fundamentally equivalent to the child's *behavioral intentions* toward smoking (e.g., 'I plan never to try a cigarette'). Intention is one of the most frequently used indices for assessing the effectiveness of anti-smoking programs, yet it is one of the most suspect measures. Not only is it obvious that intentions change and are highly situation-specific, but as we shall see shortly, children do not intend things in the same sense as adults do, and they often deny or even distort their intentions. We believe that intentions are important and useful behavior indices, but not when expressed in the abstract; only when gathered in response to actual life-like situations and dilemmas. Even so, it must be remembered that ultimately, intentions are only as stable and revealing as the underlying predispositions to view situations in consistent ways, the ability to create viable options, and to perceive, rightly or wrongly, the consequences of one's choices.

Beliefs

Traditional wisdom in the social sciences has held that beliefs exert a direct influence on actions. While we are willing to place physical health belief systems and other relevant belief systems in a causal relationship to decision-making dynamics, we question, along with other investigators, the direct causal linkage between beliefs and action. The extent to which communications influence behavior depends largely on whether or not the message is internalized by the individual. This point is well illustrated by the difference between passive acknowledgment by the general public of the message, 'Cigarette smoking causes lung cancer', and the more personalized, '*My* smoking increases *my* chances of lung cancer.' Our preliminary research indicates that the obstacles to altering or strengthening personal belief structures are formidable for several reasons. One concerns the concept of accountability; the other the developmental dynamics of intentionality.

First, many of our young interviewees represent to us that they are not smokers when, in fact, they are regular users of cigarettes. This phenomenon is more than just an effort to avoid discovery, since these children readily admit to smoking. They are not denying smoking as much as they are rejecting the label of 'smoker'. Here we see, especially in younger children, an inability to link one's personal actions with the self-attribution process. Hence, messages urging children not to 'become smokers' are often taken as being essentially addressed to someone else. The capacity for defining oneself in terms of one's behavior — in effect, accepting responsibility for one's actions — does not emerge fully until the high school years, well after the time most youngsters are exposed to smoking.

Second, in our society accountability for one's actions depends as much on one's intentions as on the gravity of the actions themselves. Thus, if a person harms another, but without intending to do so, then their culpability is diminished. Many of our young informants appear to have smoked without ever having made a conscious decision to do so. Indeed, some 12 per cent of the responses to our smoking questionnaire indicate smoking episodes without intention and without any particular thought given to them (i.e., simply because the cigarettes were available). Thus, because so often there is no intention to smoke it seems unreasonable from the adolescent viewpoint that they should suffer negative health consequences. The responsibility for smoking behavior is either attributed to others (e.g., 'the group made me do it') or is compartmentalized away from intentions. Such denial is expressed repeatedly in the smoking scenarios. Time and again, cigarettes are suddenly thrust upon the characters without consent or warning. In one teen's amusing story about smoking initiation the hapless adolescent was forced to smoke at gunpoint! Once again, these adolescents do not deny the act of smoking, only responsibility for it.

It is a truism that beliefs interact with and influence personal decisions. But before physical health messages can truly be internalized, the perceived linkage between cause and effect and personal intentionality must be strengthened. We are considering a number of strategies for achieving this objective, among them the development of *probability games* designed to simulate real-life situations and factors affecting the youngster's (player's) acceptance or rejection of smoking risks. For example, we plan to explore the possibility of fostering a life-cycle perspective that relates short-term smoking decisions to long-term consequences. This might involve a sequential series of games in which the short-term advantage of smoking in an earlier round in order to gain peer-group acceptance (in the teenage years) puts the player at a handicap in future rounds when the objective is now to establish financial independence — a task made uncertain by increased health risks, ineligibility for certain jobs, and unexpected medical expenses. Here delayed cause and effect dynamics can be discovered and the implications understood by the child without preaching from adults, and in situations that are inherently interesting.

Smoking Antecedents

Smoking behavior with all its attendant intentions, decision-making and belief structures is conditioned by a complex set of antecedent dispositions including personality, social and environmental factors. Direct attempts to engineer changes in these powerful factors are, in most cases, neither feasible nor politically acceptable. Yet anti-smoking interventions may nonetheless be designed to offset the negative aspects of a limiting environment and/or strengthen certain positive aspects. For example, increasingly research indicates that individuals who perceive themselves as responsible for their own behavior are more resistant to potentially harmful risk-behavior such as overeating and smoking. Therefore, by introducing efficacy training, possibly of the kind described in the last section, we may override a sense of personal ineffectiveness when it comes to beliefs about controlling one's health risks.

Another predisposing factor of particular interest to us, and mentioned briefly before, regards the enmeshment of individuals with social networks and with substances. The majority of our young admitted smokers perceive that it is principally *they* who make the decisions that affect their lives, whereas the preponderance of non-smokers nominate their parents and other family members for this vital role. From this evidence, we suspect that young smokers may lack a sufficient network of highly differentiated roles (e.g., 'dutiful child', 'aspiring athlete', etc.) so important in directing decisions, in encouraging trust, and in providing an orderly and stable environment. At the same time, our young smokers seem highly vigilant regarding peer group and family dynamics, appearing overly anxious to alter their allegiances to fit any changes in the power structure of the home or peer group. This perceived need to pursue shifting alignments, and the instability it creates, draws children away from a commitment to taking a stand on issues. It may lead to a frequently expressed solution theme among smokers that 'Pat (Jim) should do whatever she (he) *wants* to do.' This remark represents a simplistic abdication of judgmental processes and reflects a lack of knowing what to do, rather than indicating the most advanced levels of interpersonal reasoning in which the preferences and imperatives of the individuals are thoughtfully integrated with those of the broader social system. On the other hand, our non-smokers seem more willing: (1) to take a stance on an issue, and (2) to structure situations in ways that lead to resolutions which incidentally avoid health risks, without a loss of power or affiliation.

In closing, it is useful to summarize the essential ingredients of our intended intervention materials as they follow from our dilemma-resolution approach to health-risk behavior. Basically, our efforts will be client-centered, field-based, and developmentally realistic. They will focus on aiding individuals to manipulate their own legitimate intentions, balancing one against another in such a manner that the individual chooses a course of action that he or she perceives as a 'best possible solution'. In this way, desired motivations, intentions, and ultimately behaviors themselves will be both internalized and internally generated, thereby providing a more permanent basis for dealing with a whole range of health-risk issues.

References

LEVENTHAL, H. and CLEARY, P.D. (1980) 'The smoking problem: A review of the research and theory in behavioral risk modification', *Psychological Bulletin*, 88, pp. 370–405.

Part 3. Professional Training

Introduction

This section concentrates on professional training from two contrasting standpoints: 'national policy' and 'radical alternatives'. Hans Saan's chapter concerns the relationship between the development of school health education and training in one country, The Netherlands. Although developments in the past may have been piecemeal, school health education is now clearly on the national education map and producing specialists at both initial teacher training and in-service training levels. Although he regards training as only part of health education policy development, joint training is, nevertheless, frequently the most important vehicle for promoting a common school-community understanding. He draws upon recent work in his postgraduate training centre to illustrate criteria in assisting decision-making along the school-community boundary, i.e., stage of development of school health education, level of innovation being considered, and formal responsibilities.

Keith Tone's chapter approaches training issues via a critical view of the relationship between health education in schools and health education in the community in order to shed light on the ways in which the school might contribute most effectively to community health within an integrated community effort. A coherent programme of professional preparation for teachers of health education cannot be formulated without proper role delineation. Before this can be done it is important to recognize that fundamentally different approaches to health education may be adopted. An 'educational' approach would be concerned only to promote understanding of health issues, while a 'preventive model' would define the primary aim of health education as behaviour change. This latter approach would see the school as a branch of preventive medicine seeking to promote a healthy lifestyle in its students. A third 'radical model' would find the medical model ineffective and even unethical. The radical health educator would reject a lifestyle modification approach as mere 'victim-blaming' and would seek to persuade the school to address the social, political and economic roots of health problems. One or other of these approaches may prove to be more or less acceptable in particular cultures. In the UK, however, with its decentralized system and school-centred autonomy, different approaches may be identified not only between schools but within schools. In many schools some poorly articulated amalgam of all approaches might be deduced from analysis of formal and hidden curricula. It is argued, however, that in order to achieve the kind of *genuine* informed health decision-making to which most thoughtful health educators are likely to pay lip service, a fourth approach should be adopted — an approach which leads to self-empowerment.

Education for self-empowerment focuses on the provision of 'life skills' and involves integrated tactics designed to enhance self-esteem and promote internal locus of control. Only in this way can a school prepare its students to achieve mental, physical and social well-being in an age of 'culture shock'. Self-empowerment education demands particular and rare teaching skills. It is suggested that the most appropriate way for trainee teachers to acquire such skills is to expose them to the kinds of experiences which their future pupils will enjoy so that, for example, they clarify their own health values and acquire 'life skills'. Later through in-service training, some of them might acquire further knowledge and skills to enable them to perform the specialist functions of a health education coordinator.

A discussion of the points raised in this chapter is set out in the Appendix pp. 217–9.

Training for the School-Community Interface in Health Education

Hans Saan

Suppose you were asked to prepare two days of training on the school-community interface. Participants would expect the training to increase mutual understanding and to develop skills to cooperate effectively. One thing to be considered would be the roles of the participants in school and community. A local health authority and a chairman of a national union of teachers have different interests and would be served by different training schemes.

In this paper some variables which influence these curriculum-related decisions will be considered. Although in general these variables are described in a more abstract framework of curriculum development, the situation in The Netherlands derives from experience. Health education in The Netherlands will be the first subject of this paper; curriculum development and the school-community interface will be the second.

Health Education in The Netherlands

The Limits of This Overview

Health education can be conceived as a sub-system of health and of education systems in a society. To explain developments in the sub-system some excursions into its context are unavoidable. Even the societal environment may do more than add local colour to the picture. For The Netherlands the split into a northern part with a Calvinist tradition and a southern part with a Roman Catholic tradition has affected inhabitants' reactions to such issues as life, death, health and authority. Although this split is less pronounced than formerly, due to a general tendency away from religious affiliation, many variables could be mentioned. This paper takes a more limited approach. As earlier publications on the Dutch situation are available, here the emphasis is on education and training.

Hans Saan (Netherlands)

Developments in the 1970s

In the seventies the conditions for the development of health education were very favourable. There was a steady increase in the number of health education specialists and the quantity and quality of health education efforts increased. This development was fostered and followed by a number of reports, papers, theses, etc., which informed health education and gave it a more stable basis. The following were key developments.

1972   The report, *Health Education in Primary Schools* for the first time paid attention to health education at the primary school level.

1974   An experimental postgraduate training course for health education specialists commenced. A report on the preparation of teachers of health education in vocational training was published.

1975   Based on the 1974 report several teacher training institutes started offering professional preparation courses in health education.

1976   A National Committee on Health Education was organized to advise the Ministry of Health on a health education system, structure and finance.

1977   Dr W. Rouwenhorst prepared the first thesis on health education.

1978   Informal meetings between health educators were already customary; a Dutch Union for Health Education was founded.

1979   The Union started to publish its own bulletin. Teacher trainers organized their first National Conference on School Health Education.

1980   Full-time university training for health education specialists started at Maastricht.

1981   The Dutch National Centre for Health Education was established. The National Committee presented its final report.

There was a marked increase in all kinds of journals of topics and themes connected with health education, and there has been an increase in the availability of curriculum materials, many produced by national organizations, some theme-centred, but only a proportion based on an integrated school health education concept. With regard to legislation and policy development the picture is still diffuse: several acts relevant to health education are being discussed, but definite outcomes are still awaited.

School Health Education As a System

A systems approach to school health education helps to clarify the present situation. Figure 1 shows school and health systems as part of the

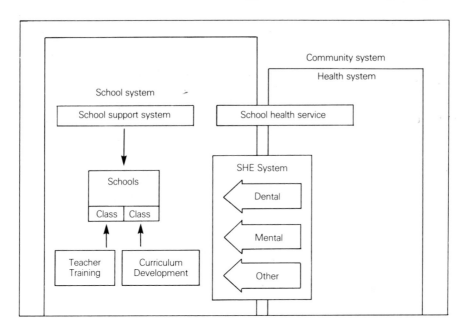

Figure 1. The School Health Education System

community system. The school health service and school health education system bridge the gap between the two. The Dutch school health service very often neglected educational opportunities and restricted itself to screening (learning) disabilities. In dental health a tradition of an integrated approach to service and education exists. Mental health education was involved mainly with sex and alcohol/drugs education. Other national organizations also took initiatives to introduce health related themes (nutrition, safety) to schools. Within the school system isolated initiatives to develop school health education also took place. Teacher training was not, like curriculum development, directed at primary schools. For secondary (vocational) training teachers are being prepared, but little teaching material is available. The school support systems sometimes interpret their role to include health education.

This haphazard development has created friction, and a clear policy is now being asked for. One problem is that many ideas on school health education were developed in a period of prosperity; we now have to adjust to a situation of decreasing resources. So the concept of school health education is being tested as to its real value and is about to show its resistance to devaluation.

Hans Saan (Netherlands)

Professional (P)reparation in School Health Education

'(P)reparation' is the term chosen here to cover both pre- and in-service training. Figure 2 gives an overview of the situation.

A distinction is made between primary and secondary education, as it is in the preparation of teachers. As a new combination of primary school and kindergarten is being considered, proposals for school health education training units are being prepared.

The training of secondary teachers on a more professional basis started only ten years ago. Nevertheless, many university courses qualify one to teach at higher levels of secondary education. New teacher training institutes qualify mainly for the lower levels. Gradually a system of in-service requalification for teachers is also developing in these new institutes. In all,

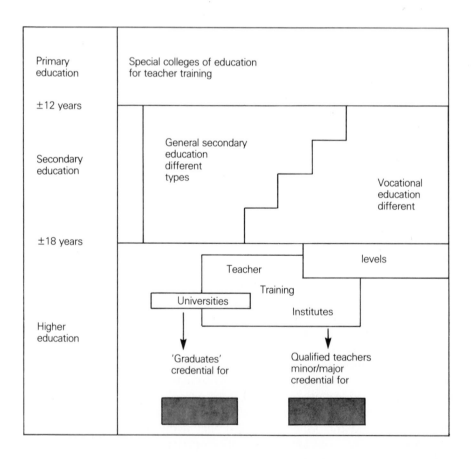

Figure 2. Professional (P)reparation in School Health Education

in seven institutes, about sixty teacher trainers produce 250–300 qualified school health education teachers a year, many more than the present number of vacancies. Some find work in community health education.

The (P)reparation of Health Education Specialists

Until 1980 no specialist preparation for health education was available. Some universities had a special interest in health education because it bordered their main field (e.g., agricultural extension education at Wageningen, human sciences at Groningen). Until then most so-called health education specialists had received only preparation in the social sciences; a few health educators were medical doctors who entered this field. Some

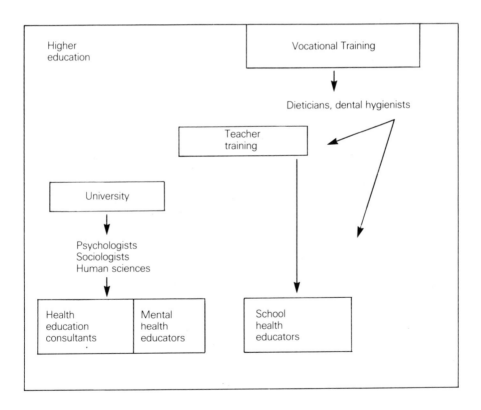

Figure 3. Professional (P)reparation in Health Education

dental hygienists, dieticians, etc. who have a health education role seldom refer to themselves as health education specialists because their traditional professional title is more commonly accepted.

Due to divisions at the governmental level we distinguish between health education, mental health education and school health education. The numbers of the last group have already been mentioned. Mental health education specialists now number about 100, but these figures are deceptive because of part-time jobs and voluntary cooperation. Health educators are still more difficult to count: the recently established union now has about 180 members, the majority of whom would call themselves health education specialists or consultants. (see Figure 3).

Postgraduate Training at the Hogere School voor Gezondheidszorg

The Hogere School voor Gezondheidszorg in Utrecht is a school of public health, involved in the training of nurses and doctors (especially doctors in social medicine). In 1974 it started the first postgraduate experimental training course in health education. Only a small part of the course was devoted to school health education: some students did an inventory on teaching methods for health education. The consultants were Warren E. Schaller and Loren B. Bensley Jr from the USA. Their presence made it possible to arrange a special workshop on school health education, which brought together many people who had seldom met before, e.g., teacher trainers (then recently appointed), curriculum developers and health education consultants.

The activities at the school can be set out as in Figure 4. Training activities are mainly directed at and based on field experience in consultation. Some examples of recent activities show that the boundaries between training, consultation and developmental support are unclear.

Definitions and concepts of school health education were studied in a workshop on 'Education and Health' (1979).
A programme comparison between all teacher training colleges was organized to develop criteria for comparison and to increase cooperation (1979).
Trefor Williams addressed a group of teacher trainers, curriculum developers and community health eductors on 'Health Education in School' via the British Schools Council Health Education Projects.

All these activities are developed in close collaboration with the participants. Sometimes the initiative for courses is taken by the school. Recent courses relevant to school health education were 'Gaming and Simulation' and 'Values Clarification'. Indirectly relevant were courses on 'Consultation' and 'Project Development'. In addition, the initial contact between health

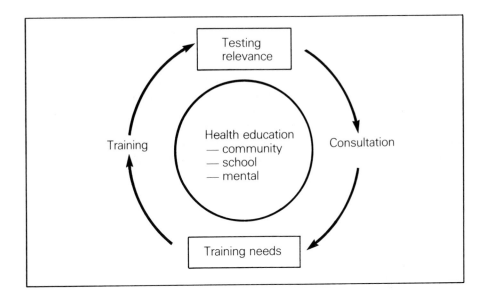

Figure 4. Activities of the Hogere School voor Gezindheidszorg

education specialists and the school system provides scope for role-play exercises. At present no formal qualification is awarded for participation in these courses.

Final Remarks

The main features of developments in recent years are:

1 the dominance of social scientists and limited cooperation with the established 'medical system';
2 the lack of coordination of health education initiatives. Too often 'accidental' decisions in one field are not connected with decisions in related fields;
3 territorial fights about health education are to be expected as many professions are overproducing manpower. Health education may become an arena of struggle among doctors, old and new health education specialists, biologists, moral developmentalists, counsellors, etc.

Hans Saan (Netherlands)

Curriculum Development and the School-Community Interface

Training, a Partial Solution

Some problems of the school-community interface can be solved by education and training. In a broad concept of systematic policy development, training is to be seen as part of the manpower selection, (p)reparation and utilization triad. Manpower, together with money, materials and methods, enables us, within a given legislatory framework and organizational context, to reach the objectives set. So it should be stressed that training can only be a partial solution to any problem. It becomes especially important in the school-health system interface because of different systems of legislation, organizational structure, professional traditions, etc.

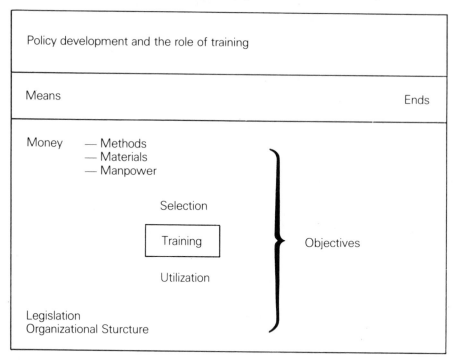

Figure 5.   The Role of Training in General Policy

Even if the partial role of training is recognized and solutions for other problems are sought, the problems that training has to solve must be specified. Two common strategies are:

1   training in health education content: 'If everyone is aware of what it is all about, cooperation will be far easier', is the rationale of this approach;

2   training in cooperation: 'If everyone is aware of problems of cooperation, negotiation, teambuilding, etc., the handling of any subject will be very easy.' This can be considered as a more general community development approach.

Most training programmes will be a combination of these two approaches. To determine the right combination, special attention should be given to the developmental stage at which health education seems to be, and to the professional roles of participants in the systems.

Developmental Stages of School Health Education

School health education has a long tradition and a short history in The Netherlands. Three stages can be identified in its development.

Stage I.   Disease warnings   In many schools 'disease education' has been (and sometimes is still) dominant. The main characteristics are:

> legitimation by society's disquiet on some subjects (sex, drugs, etc.),
> this causes the school to invite an expert (quick service),
> to give objective information based on scientific models,
> concluding with some popular warnings and simple messages.

Associated with this approach are usually:

> no coordination between school, experts, themes, messages, etc.,
> raised index-finger as the most important instrument,
> motto: 'do as I say, don't do as I do.'

Stage II.   Pioneers of health education   Partly as a reaction to stage I, newly appointed health education experts (over)stimulate their audience, with the followings characteristics:

> preferably invited rather than imposed upon schools,
> personal competence as a central theme,
> group discussion as a major instrument,
> development of material starts incidentally,
> legitimation is mainly by a non-disease, life-centred, responsibility-centred approach,
> close cooperation with some teachers,

As this is a pioneer stage, other features are:

> same names appear everywhere,
> simple innovation models are based on trial, error and personal preference,
> there is a short time perspective,
> effectiveness is limited, with little active dissemination of experience.

Stage III.   Systems start to develop   As feedback on materials, manpower, policy development, etc. increases, school health education moves away from the incidental to the systematic:

> legitimation is increasingly based on legislation and regulation,
> organizations take over responsibilities from the pioneers,
> innovation is by multiple models,
> many are involved, and roles are continually revised (e.g., school health service),
> the time perspective is enlarged,
> there is a reintegration of a disease perspective (e.g., in patient education, self-help) in competence-enhancing approaches.

The developmental stages can be seen in combination as in Figure 6. The relevance of this three-stage model for the development of training is mainly in selection of relevant objectives. The actual situation in a community reflects a certain stage, and the decision to develop skills relevant to this stage or to foster transition to the next stage is crucial. In terms of the two strategies mentioned above, *content* would probably be dominant: i.e., what do we expect health education in school to be?

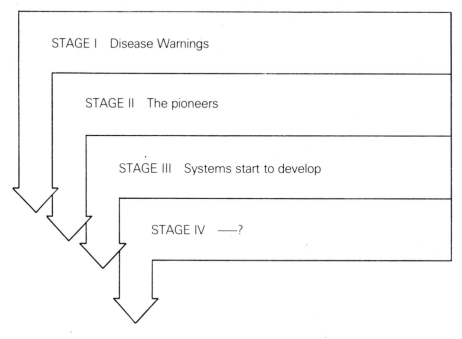

Figure 6.   Developmental Stages in Health Education

Health Education As an Innovation in the School System

The introduction of health education in the school system has features of innovation in an organization. The scope of the change determines how many are involved and in what roles they will participate.

It is useful to distinguish three process levels of innovation:

1 *The classroom.* In the classroom one teacher is mainly responsible for selection of content and method and for interpretation of the teacher's role. The key question is how far the personalization of health eduction should go or whether a more detached 'objective' presentation is required.

2 *The school.* The headteacher and/or the team have to answer classroom-specific questions, but also more general questions such as how do we integrate health in the total curriculum? does this have consequences for subjects, pupil groupings, the timetable, etc.? does it require team teaching, outside resources, outsiders to participate, etc? which question leads to:

3 *School-community.* how do we organize our relations with outsiders? who is responsible? who pays? how to continue cooperation? (procedures, roles, rules, etc.).

The range of questions is very broad, and it is important that training takes into account the present role and level of responsibility of those involved. Training should help to solve level-specific problems and treat other levels as illuminating conditions or contexts. The problems are, in general, more of an organizational nature, and solutions depend heavily on the readiness and mutual trust of participants. Dominant is the question: how do we expect to cooperate?

Practical Consequences for Training

Decisions for training on content and cooperation are not independent. The simple matrix in Figure 7 shows the most frequent combination. In several Dutch projects the systems stage is achieved by a very careful pooling of incidental experience among several classes in some schools in cooperation with many 'outsiders'.

In-service training for these projects is now mainly directed at the 'intake' point of first contact with the school system. Many teachers are leaving the disease approach and looking for alternatives. However, it would be unwise in a first contact to 'jump a stage' and try to move from class-level change to systems development over all. This would not only overstep the formal roles of those involved, it would also go beyond their perception of what is relevant.

Levels of change	Stages of development		
	Disease	Pioneer	Systems
Class	+	+	+
School	−	+	+
School-community	−	−	+

Figure 7. Stages and Levels Combined

These models are mainly helpful for trainers assessing realistic objectives. It is essential to become aware of differences in expectations and motivation when starting health education in schools.

Approaches to Professional Training in Health Education

Keith Tones

The purpose of this chapter is to consider approaches to professional training. It will not, however, provide an ideal or model curriculum for colleges and departments of education: this would prove tedious and unrealistic. Nor will it review the current status of professional training in the United Kingdom and its very real inadequacies. However, it will attempt to look critically at the relationship between health education in schools and health education within the community; it will examine the compatibility of different approaches and above all consider ways in which the school might contribute most effectively to community health within the context of an integrated community effort. The importance of pursuing the goal of self-empowerment will be emphasized. Only then will consideration be given to implications for the professional education and training of teachers who will undoubtedly have to overcome considerable barriers of inertia and even hostility. Health educators will have to tackle a major programme of innovation if schools are to fulfil their potential contribution to the mental, physical and social health of society.

Approaches to Health Education in School and Community

An argument has already been made elsewhere for an integrated approach to health education which involves both school and the wider community.[1] However, before integration is possible, it is important to recognize and clarify different philosophical and ethical stances which might otherwise hinder such collaborative efforts. It is useful to identify four major approaches to health education[2] and while there may well be overlap between such approaches, there are certain fundamental differences in emphasis which, if not subjected to critical scrutiny, may cloud discussion and lead to unproductive debate. Indeed, it might be argued that failure to clarify aims and approaches may result in abortive programmes within a school or community health education service.

Education and Prevention

The first distinction is between an 'educational' and a 'preventive' approach. The first of these is, superficially at least, particularly relevant to the practice of health education in schools, while the second might seem to be the prerogative of a community health education service. An educational approach is primarily concerned with the delivery of knowledge. In its most refined and educationally sound form it would involve not merely the supply information but the adoption of strategies to ensure that information had been understood, relevant beliefs and values had been clarified and opportunities had been provided for the practice of decision-making in simulated settings. According to this approach no pressures should be placed on the individual to make a particular 'healthy' decision. The educational task is concerned to foster 'informed decision-making'. Success is measured in terms of completeness of understanding rather than attitude change or behavioural outcome. Schools — particularly in Europe — are traditionally concerned with this type of function. Indeed, emphasis is often placed only on the first stage — the acquisition of information.

If, on the other hand, we consider the conventional community health service approach, it is clear that such goals as 'understanding' or 'informed choice' would be very much secondary to a direct preventive function. In fact a teacher might be successful in promoting informed decision-making of a kind which a physician might well consider to have been counterproductive insofar as it did not lead to a preventive outcome. It is of course well established that knowledge does not necessarily lead to action and since behaviour is intimately related to both the aetiology and management of current health problems in western societies, it is clear that health education, in the context of a medical model, will have as its goal the modification of behaviours in order to prevent those diseases which contemporary medicine finds it difficult or impossible to cure. There can be little doubt that the medical profession will view the schools as an arm of preventive medicine — a fact attested to by several recent government reports.[3] However, it would be wrong to give the impression that teachers wholeheartedly support the 'educational model' and a survey by Rossington demonstrated that teachers had mixed views about the matter — or in many cases had apparently not even thought about it![4] Equally it would be incorrect to assume that community health educators always espouse a persuasive-preventive approach. SOPHE has apparently subscribed to the doctrine of 'informed choice',[5] a view supported by Green, who defined health education as '... any combination of learning opportunities designed to facilitate **voluntary** adaptation of behaviour which will improve or maintain health.'[6]

It is nonetheless important for teachers to examine this issue and grapple with the dilemma arising from the fact that few people are in a position to make a genuinely informed choice about the behaviours they adopt. This is especially important since it may well be that the school alone is in a position to stimulate preventive actions — a fact well illustrated by the case of site-specific cancer education. The main thrust of this kind of preventive programme is to promote understanding of the significance of the so-called 'seven warning signs and symptoms of cancer' and to motivate people to seek early medical advice whenever one of these symptoms is experienced. Since health education programmes operating through pamphleteering and the media are likely to generate in many people anxiety and aversion which will in turn make it less likely that early diagnosis will be sought, it is difficult to see how progress might be made without a school programme. Such a programme would aim both to teach about the significance of physiological deviations from normality and reduce cancerophobia by generating realistic beliefs about cause and the effectiveness of early treatment. It would of course require skilled and sensitive teaching and a properly integrated spiral curriculum in both cognitive and affective domains.

It is worth noting in passing that adopting a preventive approach as the raison d'être of health education in schools is a risky business. In the first instance we would need to be sure that teachers had at their disposal the methodological techniques which would enable them to modify children's present and future lifestyles in the face of the powerful programming provided by primary socialization. Moreover, assuming that sufficiently powerful (and ethical) methods were available, we would need to be reasonably sure about what constituted a healthy lifestyle: epidemiological doubts and uncertainties about many contemporary health issues would suggest caution.

Involving the Home

Whether or not a preventive goal is adopted, it is difficult to see how health education may be fully effective without the involvement of the home and community. It might be argued, for example, that teachers should be concerned to modify parental behaviour either directly or indirectly by using the pupil as a change agent in an outreach programme directed at parents. Such an approach might be especially effective in smoking cessation programmes. Even if teachers are less macchiavellian, they must surely take account of culture clash. The school's teaching — especially in the affective area — is likely to make relatively little impact in competition with the often 'unhealthy' culture of the home and the 'parallel' curriculum offered by society and local community. Health education in such circumstances as these is likely to be at best ineffective and at worst may generate dissonance and anxiety in the child. Since schools are almost by definition middle-class institutions, the major clash will be with the home environment of children from lower socio-economic classes. It is hardly necessary to reiterate that the major contribution to community ill health is made by this particular 'disadvantaged' sub-culture. Any contribution by the school to community health must therefore be judged by its effectiveness in handling the health of this sector of the population. It may thus be necessary for teachers to develop and refine the notion of the community school and involve themselves in community development work along with health professionals. Any such involvement with the community would demand not only awareness of the culture of disadvantaged groups and their problems but also the acquisition of empathy and specific social skills which would allow teachers to communicate effectively. It will be clear from later comments that such training may benefit, directly or indirectly, the schoolchildren in their charge.

Radical Health Education

Increasing awareness of the need for a radical approach is discernible in health education. This may range from attempts to tackle health problems at source by, for example, pressuring government to be less weak-minded with commercial interests, to much more radical ventures stemming from observations such as Draper's that western capitalist society is inherently unhealthy: the unbridled pursuit of economic growth is accompanied by ill health; the pursuit of a healthy ecosystem is economically unproductive.[7]

Teachers must learn to tackle these aspects of the parallel curriculum and acquire not only awareness of the politics of health but also skill in treading the tightrope of political education. Any such involvement will be labelled by many as subversive and non-educational, yet it is difficult to see how 'radical' health education can be ignored by school health educators. Furthermore, there are even more radical implications to be derived from the fourth and final approach to health education, an approach which may prove to be the most effective and ethical way in which the school might tackle community health. This involves 'self-empowering' students. It poses particular training requirements.

Self-Empowerment, Health Education and the School

A narrowly preventive approach to health education will be unacceptable to many — with its epidemiological uncertainty and implications of coercion and manipulation. On the other hand, it would be naive to assume that merely discussing health issues or providing information will be sufficient to foster the informed decision-making which is the hallmark of ethical health education. Genuine freedom of choice is illusory without self-empowerment. The promotion of self-empowerment should be a major goal of health education in schools.

The notion of self-empowerment is most readily understood by considering the factors which impede an individual's freedom to choose a healthy (or unhealthy) lifestyle. These factors derive, directly or indirectly, from the social environment in which the individual finds himself and which has contributed to his socialization. The de-powering effects of cultural deprivation and the 'inner-city syndrome' need no further explanation. The lack of 'healthy' options and the presence of negative models of smoking, alcohol abuse and poor dietary practice in social class V environments are well documented. What is less obvious perhaps is the way in which the powerlessness engendered by the environment becomes internalized and imposes limits on the individual's health choices. Not only does he learn to attach little value to health generally and acquire negative attitudes to many more specific health practices, but he is also unlikely to develop a belief in his capacity to control his destiny and few skills to help him to do so. The self-empowered person, however, is more likely to possess high 'internal locus of control';[8] in other words, he is likely to have developed a firm conviction that he is not controlled by fate or by powerful others. According to Phares, 'internals':[9]

1 have greater self-control;
2 have superior academic achievement;
3 are more socially responsible;
4 are more likely to delay gratification.

It is clear that these characteristics have many important, albeit indirect, implications for health education — for instance, high academic achievers are less likely to smoke; self-control and the capacity to delay immediate gratification will predispose an individual to accept and heed health education messages promising future health to those who shun pleasurable but unhealthy behaviours. Wallston and Wallston offer evidence of more direct associations between locus of control and health.[10]

In addition to internality, the self-empowered individual will enjoy high self-esteem. This is a correlate of internality and achievement and associated with the receipt of nurturance, respect and independence training. An individual high in self-esteem will not only be more mentally healthy (by definition), but will also be better able to resist pressures and, presumably, be more receptive to health education which invites people to look after themselves.

A third component of self-empowerment is the possession of social skills. These include not only the more general skills such as assertiveness — necessary for dealing with a hostile environment — but the more specific skills involved, for example, in refusing a cigarette. The acquisition of social interaction skills will not only enhance self-esteem, but will increase internality — whcih in turn will boost self-esteem and facilitate the expression of assertiveness and relating skills.

The implications of self-empowerment for promoting mental and physical health have been discussed above. The implications for social health are even greater. We are currently observing a process of escalating unemployment which will provide a fundamental challenge to such basic social values as the work ethic. Its implications for self-esteem and for mental and physical health do not need spelling out. Non-employment is but one feature of the general phenomenon described by Toffler as future shock'.[11] Probably the most important task facing school health and social education today is that of providing anticipatory guidance to enable children to cope with 'future shock'. Hopson and Scally argue forcibly that such anticipatory guidance may be provided by 'Lifeskills Teaching'. The following lifeskills are relevant to a self-empowerment approach to health education.[12]

> how to discover my values and beliefs
> how to be positive about myself
> how to cope with and gain from life transitions
> how to be proactive
> how to cope with stress
> how to develop and use my political awareness
> how to maximize my leisure opportunities
> how to make, keep and end a relationship
> how to give and get help
> how to be assertive
> how to influence people and systems
> how to work in groups

Several health education programmes are available which seek to foster self-esteem and clarify health values, and detailed materials have been produced which aim to develop personal attributes and provide practice in social skills.[13] However, we might, with some justification, ask whether teachers are willing and able to develop lifeskills teaching and adopt a self-empowerment approach to health education. Self-empowerment teaching requires educational risk-taking — and skills which few teachers possess. At a time when, in the UK, there is little opportunity to provide coherent and comprehensive health education training for teachers, there is paradoxically an urgent need for a new approach to professional preparation.

Professional Preparation of Teachers for Health Education

The aim of this paper is not to produce a scheme of work for the preparation of teachers for the important task of health education. However, it is not difficult to provide brief specifications for such a programme if the self-empowerment approach is to be adopted.

Initial teacher education should provide:

1 an understanding of health and of contemporary (and future) health problems;
2 an understanding of major issues in school health education practice;
3 a values and belief clarification exercise about students' own health;
4 a programme of lifeskills teaching designed to self-empower the students;
5 skills in affective teaching, including face-to-face relating skills and group teaching skills.

In-service courses should aim to provide an opportunity to reassess issues and to provide mature and experienced teachers with the further specialist knowledge and skills necessary to enable them to coordinate health and social education activities across the curriculum. Hopefully, by dint of employing the self-empowerment skills acquired during initial training, they will have risen to a position of pre-eminence within the school and will have persuaded the headteacher to institute a comprehensive and coherent integrated programme of health and social education for them to coordinate.

Notes

1 TONES, B.K. (1976) 'The organization of community health education: A case for strategic integration', *Health Education*, September/October, pp. 16–19.
2 TONES, B.K. (1981) 'Health education: Prevention or subversion?', *Royal Society of Health Journal*, 3, pp. 114–7
3 See, for instance, SELECT COMMITTEE ON VIOLENCE IN THE FAMILY (1974–75) *'Violence in Marriage'*, London, HMSO; BRITISH NUTRITION FOUNDATION, DHSS and the HEALTH EDUCATION COUNCIL (1977) *Nutrition Education*, London, HMSO; COMMITTEE ON CHILD HEALTH SERVICES (1977) *'Fit for the Future*, Vol. 1, London, HMSO.
4 ROSSINGTON, R. (1975) Unpublished MSc. Thesis, Department Community Health, University of Manchester.
5 GREEN, L.W. (1978) 'Determining the impact and effectiveness of health education as it relates to federal policy', *Health Education Monographs*, 6 (Suppl.), pp. 28–66.
6 SOCIETY FOR PUBLIC HEALTH EDUCATION (1976) *'Code of Ethics'* 15 October, 1976, San Francisco, Calif.
7 DRAPER, P. (1977) 'Health and wealth', *Royal Society of Health Journal*, June.
8 ROTTER, J.B. (1966) 'Generalised expectancies for internal versus external control of reinforcement'. *Psy. Monographs*, 80, 1.
9 PHARES, J.E. (1976) *Locus of Control in Personality*, New Jersey, General Learning Press.
10 WALLSTON, K.A. and WALLSTON, B.S. (Eds) (1978) 'Health locus of council', *Health Education Monographs*, 6, 2, Spring.
11 TOFFLER, A. (1970) Future Shock, London, Bodley Head.
12 HOPSON, B. and SCALLY, M. (1981) *'Lifeskills Teaching'*, London, McGraw Hill.

Keith Tones (UK)

13 SCHOOLS COUNCIL (1976) '*Schools Council Health Education Project 5–13*', London, Nelson; MCPHAIL, P. (1977) *Living Well*, London, Longmans; BUTTON, L. (1974) *Developmental Group Work with Adolescents*, London, Hodder and Stoughton; BALDWIN, J. and WELLS, H. (1979) *Active Tutorial Work, Books 1–4*, Oxford, Blackwell; HOPSON, B. and SCALLY, M. (1981) *Lifeskills Teaching Programmes No. 1*, Leeds, Lifeskills Associates.

Part 4. Cooperative Health Education: Ideas and Initiatives

Introduction

The purpose of Part 4 is to present examples of cooperative health education occurring among different professional groups and agencies in selected areas of health education not covered in the earlier chapters, and particularly from those countries not represented in the same chapters. Some of the examples are more advanced in terms of projects realized than others where the innovation may not have progressed beyond the planning stage. The following chapters therefore represent a range of achievement in key areas of health education where success depends upon a high degree of intergroup cooperation, and to a large extent they mark progress in those problem areas highlighted at the Seminar.

In 'The Role of School Health Services in School Health Education Programmes' Lea Maes describes recent development projects in Belgium, Sweden, Switzerland and the USA, and outlines current constraints. She identifies four main tasks for school health services: (1) to provide basic information; (2) to integrate health education elements in periodic health or medical examinations of pupils; (3) to provide learning and training opportunities in first aid and dental care; (4) to provide information on medical aspects of health education programmes. Unlike other chapters in Part 4 which post-date the Seminar, Lea Maes' paper was discussed in detail at the Seminar. The main points of this discussion appear on page 221.

In the paper entitled 'From the Screening of Illnesses to Psycho-Social Support for Schoolchildren' Matti Rimpelä reviews the changing epidemiology of Finland and demonstrates the need for closer interagency cooperation, as psycho-social problems replace more traditional disease patterns. However, in a country as well attuned to such complex 'diseases of civilization' as cardiovascular disease the interdependence of the psycho-social and the physical is fully appreciated and new national regulations provide a statutory basis for promoting discussion about these matters among interested parties. Hopefully this will lead to increased, purposeful community action which ought to include strong persuasion to revise the initial teacher training curriculum which at present does not adequately prepare teachers for their health education task.

'Oral and Dental Hygiene at School' by Colette Menard sets out some recent initiatives in dental health education in French schools and communities. These have been at national, regional and local levels, and have involved health policy-makers and administrators, school and community health personnel, dentists, parents and children. The work has been carefully evaluated and while significant progress has been made, the way is clear for new initiatives.

In 'Health Education and the Environment in the Basic School Curriculum in Norway', Arne Hauknes outlines the way in which curricular legislation has paved the way for important developments in health education for all age groups which includes back-up roles of school health service personnel. Health education is seen in terms of not just an individual's responsibility for himself but also for the community in the widest sense. It starts at the point that makes the deepest impact, the immediate environment, which is viewed both physically and socially. In the example 'Smoking and Health', the methodology is comprehensive, embracing the acquisition and assimilation of knowledge, and development of understanding, attitudes and skills, and has been carefully piloted and evaluated. Teachers involve parents and other members of the community in the work.

In 'The Multicultural Background to Health Education', Mary Holmes summarizes the findings of a small feasibility study she conducted on behalf of the Department of Education and Science in the United Kingdom. After outlining some of the difficulties faced by minority groups in the community and by those who teach the children, she outlines a broad strategy based on recognition of the positive contribution minority groups can make to the cultural enrichment of the nation through education. She concludes with suggestions for practical measures in the school curriculum.

Herbert D. Thier in 'Using Science and Health Teaching to Enable the Disabled' sets out a strategy for assisting the disabled to become full members of society. Scientific literacy and the ability to collect, evaluate, and use evidence as the basis for one's decision-making are cultural imperatives for any participating member of a free society. Whether deciding which of similar items is a better buy at the supermarket, interpreting advertizing and its claims in regard to one's own health or well-being, or making major decisions as a voter on environmental or other major issues, the individual needs the ability to collect and analyze the evidence in order to make a reasonable decision. This is why an effective science programme which teaches these skills is a necessity for all learners, disabled or not. The science programme, in addition, can have a significant effect in helping disabled individuals to maximize their capabilities while minimizing their disabilities, leading to greater independence and self-reliance. An independent, self-reliant disabled individual can be a fully contributing member of the society. The alternative is the totally dependent individual who has to be cared for indefinitely at costs per year far in excess of the entire cost of providing an effective science and health programme. Science and health education cannot solve all problems, but they can make a significant contribution.

In 'A Programme of Nutritional Education in Outlying Areas of Spain with a High Incidence of Goitre' Pilar Najera outlines the nature and origins of a problem not uncommon in isolated areas and then sets out policies, strategies and methods to overcome it. She describes the implementation of a carefully planned and coordinated programme involving members of the public, manufacturers, shopkeepers, the media and education, health and medical agencies. The programme is still in its early stages but the evaluation so far is positive.

In 'Health Education and Initial Teacher Training in England and Wales' Trefor Williams reviews progress of the project team which he directs in determining possible strategies, methods and materials for those involved in the preparation of school teachers. The three main preparatory phases were: (1) a national survey of schools, (2) a national survey of initial teacher education courses; and (3) a national study of the students. The findings which are summarized have contributed substantially to identifying and clarifying potentially productive courses of action which are set out in the 'plan for action'.

In 'Trial Interprofessional Workshop Courses in School and Community Health Education', George Campbell summarizes the independent evaluation of a series of in-service courses of an innovative nature conducted by a voluntary organization, the Family Planning Association, in the United Kingdom. Their special features included work in a highly sensitive area of the curriculum: sexuality and personal relationships education, recruitment of a representative group of different health, medical and educational personnel from particular schools and their catchment areas, and an experiential basis to their learning through carefully graded workshop exercises. The evaluation indicated that the stated aims and objectives were achieved. Furthermore, a potentially highly effective model suitable for adaptation in other topic areas of health education.

While the chapters in Part 4 represent new ideas and initiatives in six European countries and the USA they are not by any means the whole picture of development but merely examples selected by those who took part in the original Seminar. What is important, however, is the extent to which the work outlined faces the issues and answers the questions raised at the Seminar.

Of the constraints identified, analyzed and discussed in Part I the most important were 'boundary issues'. Most of the chapters in Part 4 take up this challenge in that those concerned with initiatives at the national level (in Finland, France, Norway and Spain) have anticipated problems between the different levels of authority, i.e., national, regional and local. In addition, the need for varied professional and lay involvement has meant the overcoming of some traditional and counterproductive ways of working, not without raising further problems, not least that of continuing communication if cooperative work is to be sustained. Space does not allow the inclusion of all the methods employed to achieve collaboration, although Campbell outlines one potentially productive learning approach being employed on an increasing scale in the UK, Western Europe and North America.

However enlightened and potentially effective the local initiative, if the overall strategy is not in harmony, the local initiative will founder. For this reason it is important to underline the need for higher-level support (national or regional) even though an initiative may start at a lower level (regional or local). If there is a national or regional policy and strategy this will lend weight to a local experiment or innovation and facilitate development. This is particularly true where finance is needed and may be forthcoming from a higher authority, say for pump-priming a particular innovation. Unfortunately, some higher-level support is not matched by effective back-up lower down; at worst this becomes mere lip-service to an innovation. In the paper on trial interprofessional workshops, Campbell reports consultation and agreement at the planning stage with policy-makers and administrative officers, and yet effective support at the later stages of recruitment and attendance varied considerably, which adversely affected the work.

Where national government is strongly counterbalanced by regional or local government, as in most countries of Western Europe and North America, policies and priorities may be viewed differently and nationally inspired initiatives may be frustrated at lower levels, the degree depending on the powers invested in regional or local government and their financial independence. One feature in western democratic countries where political power is decentralized is differential or piecemeal development. Most of the chapters in Part 4 reveal signs of this. On the other hand, effective local or regional government can enable a lead to be given through an innovation to which national government is either hostile or at best luke-warm. At a time when objectives are seen increasingly by financially hard-pressed national governments in economic and cost-effective terms in the short-term, a regional or local stand on health education objectives and practice with longer-term beneficial results may be essential in spite of the formidable difficulties.

One of the dangers of local initiatives is that unless there is good communication with regional and national bodies, news of a successful experiment or development may be lost to the outside world. In this respect it is important to note that while 'the trial interprofessional workshop courses' of Chapter 16 were proposed by a local education officer the fact that she was employed by the Family Planning Association, a national organization currently engaged in experimenting with new 'training the trainer' methods, meant automatically a wider circle of interest and wider dissemination of results through their national network. The same is true of local initiatives in school health education linked to the UK Schools Council Health Education Projects.

Health education poses a special problem in that it requires the collaboration of two key services — health and education — if it is to be fully informed and effective, and able to draw upon relevant resources. This is not easy to achieve in practice for while both services may see the need to work together, their differing perspectives on what health education is, what the objectives (goals) should be, what methods are appropriate, and how programmes should be evaluated, may prevent it. This in addition to the problem that busy people have of finding the time to meet together at regular intervals, for a purpose that while seen to be important may not have the urgency or priority of some of the more pressing immediate problems of, for example, maintaining a viable service for their clients.

Inevitably, the lead is taken by one service, either health or education, which recognizes the importance of pursuing a deliberate policy. The UK is a patchwork reflecting local variations in initiatives taken. But for successful implementation it is necessary for the two services to work together. In those parts of the UK where health education in school seems to have taken root such partnerships appear to be more firmly grounded.

Although evidence from work in France (Menard) and Norway (Hauknes) supports the general observation that boundaries are more permeable at primary school level than at secondary, the fact that several countries are engaging in the more intractable problems of older pupils, where school-community links are less developed, is all the more encouraging. The key role of the parent is being increasingly recognized for all age groups. This, in turn, is closely linked to that other constraint, 'the practical difficulties of involving clients in the identification of their own needs and priorities.' Clearly, the involvement of parents could help bridge the gap between teachers and pupils where family beliefs and attitudes are often the starting point for new learning opportunities. However, the problem of isolated, shy, uneducated or inarticulate parents remains acute, and is bound to hinder the progress of the health education of their children where there may be no consensus between home and school. The slow progress in health education of children of various ethnic minorities and handicapped children in Western Europe and North America is a testimony to this, as the chapters by Holmes and Thier indicate.

The philosophy of health education and health promotion implicit in the models presented in several of the following chapters focuses on the individual level; it is not only about 'self-help' but about one-self as a member of a community with a responsibility for caring for others in that community whether they be close friends in the same class in school, or members of a wider international community, who may be disabled or deprived, and whom the individual may never have seen. Thus a community health education orientation, as opposed to a purely individualistic one, would appear to be gaining ground.

The Role of School Health Services in School Health Education Programmes

Lea Maes

Ideally, the purpose of school health programmes is to promote, preserve and restore the health and functional capacity of pupils. This purpose is achieved by:

1 providing optimal physical and social environmental and educational conditions;
2 promoting healthful behaviour through health education in its broadest sense, and
3 providing school health services for the early detection of disease and impairment and for the comprehensive treatment of those health problems which can be dealt with only in close connection with the school situation.[1]

These activities are the responsibility of several persons and institutions: school health services, school psychologists, headteachers, teachers, other school and community personnel, pupils and parents. Ideally, school health education programmes should involve all agencies in the school environment, with all agencies actively seeking a role. This broad school health programme is the context in which we should analyze the role of school health services in school health education programmes.

Conflicts present in existing school health services reflect a search for new structures and tasks; and health education is seen as one of the important tasks. A brief description is given below of the structure and organization of school health services to clarify the relationship to school health education programmes. Based on this outline and against the background of experimental health education activities of school health services, possible roles in school health education programmes will be formulated. Finally, the constraints and obstacles to the realization of these health education tasks will be discussed.

Lea Maes (Belgium)

Structure and Organization of School Health Services

In looking for a place for school health services in school health education programmes, everything depends on one's definition of school health services. Their structure and organization are different in each country. Differences exist in the location of school health services (in or outside the school), in people working there (only medical personnel or also social workers and psychologists), in methods of payment (per head or for a certain package of activities), in legally imposed tasks and duties, etc. All these elements can have an impact on health education activities. Nonetheless, although differences exist, the main tasks and orientations are similar. These are the basis for further discussion. As an example the structure and organization of school health services in Belgium will be outlined.

Organization and Structure of School Health Services in Belgium

In Belgium there are separate health service systems for public and private schools. For the public sector medical aspects are integrated in psycho-medico-social centres; for the private sector there are separate medical school health services.

School health services in the private sector. The 1964 law on school health services charges these services with the following tasks:

> detection of mental and physical problems in schoolchildren;
> detection of contagious diseases by educational, adminstrative and other personnel in schools;
> carrying out of preventive measures if contagious diseases are detected;
> cooperation in the drawing up of statistics on the health status of pupils;
> improvement of hygiene in schools.

These tasks are executed by accredited teams in accredited centres. Each centre consists of a doctor, a nurse, sometimes a social worker and a secretary. Periodically all schoolchildren are examined by such a team whose members are paid according to the amount of work they do. In practice, therefore, these services are characterized by quick, mass screening for urgent health problems.

In many countries, including Belgium, systematic preventive health care for schoolchildren goes back to the first half of the twentieth century,[2] when most health problems were the result of low nutrition and infection. Modern medicine and improvements in hygiene have changed totally the problem profile of schoolchildren who are now confronted with such problems as accidents, risk behaviour and emotional adaptation to school requirements.[3] The working methods of the health services are not, on the whole, adapted to coping with these new problems.

Psycho-medical-social services (PMS) in the public sector. The 1962 law charges these services with the following tasks:

> advising parents on the findings of various professionals with regard to pupils in their last year of primary school;
> examining pupils who have study problems;
> psychological, social and medical screening of all pupils;
> cooperation over research concerning the way school health knowledge is assimilated.

These tasks are executed by a team of two psychologists, a nurse or social worker and a doctor. Periodically they see all schoolchildren. Although these services have other functions, they are geared mainly towards individual guidance. The PMS services are experimenting with preventive mental health programmes to assist the work of teachers.

The Present Situation with Respect to Health Education and School Health Services

Learning about health is a complex process that starts very early, in the pre-school phase. In this first phase the family is very important; the first internalization of values and attitudes take place within the family. This is primary socialization. The school, which is an important agent of secondary socialization, must take account of the results of this primary socialization. No child that comes into school is a *tabula rasa* of health attitudes and health knowledge. The task of the school consists, first, in bringing mostly unconscious health knowledge and attitudes to the level of consciousness, and, secondly, in guiding children in their choice of rational and conscious health behaviour. This process demands continuous guidance, in which formal and informal education are not seen as contradictory, but mutually supportive. When we look at the structure, organization and work of school health services in this light, two aspects stand out as important:

1 school health services are basically a medical matter, because of the people working there and the kind of activities carried out. In practice this means that they are individual, and disease or problem-oriented. This has consequences for health education activities which are geared mostly towards individuals and specific topics;

2 school health services have only sporadic contact with the schools or pupils. This means that truly educational activities which require continuity of contact are not possible.

Lea Maes (Belgium)

Health Education Experiments in School Health Services in Four Countries

In several countries school health services are experimenting with school health education programmes. The experiments described below were chosen because they exemplify four important health educational tasks of school health services.

Belgium[4]

Health education experiments in some Belgian school health services are based on the idea of integrating health education activities with the normal periodic health examinations of schoolchildren.

In a study of the 'Alliance Nationale des Mutualités Chrétiennes' the educational significance of school health examinations was defined as follows: (1) reinforcement and legitimation of existing knowledge about health matters relevant to the age group, and (2) development of a positive attitude towards school health services in particular and preventive services in general. The learning objectives were defined as follows: children should learn the 'why' and 'how' of the examination, feel at ease while being examined and be able to participate in the procedures. The underlying aim was the development of a positive attitude vis-à-vis the school health service. The second objective was that children should get an opportunity during the examination to learn about health values and preventive measures, the underlying aim being that school health services have a reinforcing and legitimizing role in health learning.

What specifically should be looked at to operationalize these objectives? The study analyzed and defined functions and tasks of persons who could be or were important to the success of overall school health examination objectives, in particular to the educational objectives. In the school health service they identified: the child, health personnel, teachers and parents. To realize their objectives a new procedure for examining the child was set up. This contains the same tests for screening for physical and mental defects as the usual procedure, and the same health team assumes responsibility for both types of examination. The main difference consists of spreading different elements of the examination over time and making use of potential links between school and health centre system. The new examination procedure consists of three phases:

Phase 1. This starts in school one month before the examination. The teacher assumes responsibility for three preparatory lessons on the 'why' and 'how' of the periodic school health examinations and on preventive advice relative to nutrition and hygiene. Implicit in this preparatory phase is the notion that a school health examination is a special event for the child for which he or she should be prepared by the health centre team with the assistance of volunteer teachers. In addition to special lessons about the school health examination, children fill out a form where they check their health practices (sleeping, hygiene, nutrition). The underlying idea is that children will learn to think about their health in a specific way. The data also provide a practical basis for promoting communication between health staff and the child.

Phase 2.   This phase contains activities specifically designed for the waiting room, for biometric testing at the health centre and for clinical examination with the physician. The waiting room is an area where not much is being attempted apart from the reading of comics. In the new approach health games are played during waiting time. They are intended to repeat and reinforce the preparatory lessons previously taught in class. Health games have the advantage of being particularly well suited to the psychological (extra-curricular) and practical demands of the situation (children going back and forth between waiting room and examination room). At the same time they help the children feel at ease and contribute to a positive feeling about the health centre.

While the child is being prepared in class and in the waiting room for more active participation during the examinations, a special mechanism was introduced during biometrical and clinical examinations: a child-oriented record. This is a card where the child himself notes the test results (e.g., I measure 1 m 30 cm, I weigh 30 kg., I should brush my teeth after meals and at least once a day). The activity of writing implies active participation. In addition it requires the health team to communicate clearly and to work at a level of comprehension and speed of a 10-year-old.

Phase 3.   The last phase is completed in the classroom about three weeks after the examinations have taken place. The teacher discusses the children's reactions to the examination and uses the data on the child-oriented record for a lesson on growth, weight and preventive care. To relate these activities to regular classroom activities, a twenty-point knowledge test on the school health service and on prevention has been prepared for use by the teacher. It serves at the same time as a knowledge-based evaluation.

The new approach to school health examinations was developed with the understanding that no extra funds would be available and that the approach would have to be applicable to other age groups. This necessitated examination of the same number of children in experimental or control conditions without changes or additions to staff. There was no money for over-time. The only cost was in the production of lesson plans, health games and paperwork for the project.

The main problem is that the new examination procedures require more attention and intensive involvement of staff with the child, which is more satisfying for staff and child, but also more mentally and physically exhausting.

It is the general opinion of staff that the new approach cannot, under present constraints of time and money, be extended to all age groups if priorities and the administrative framework of the school health service are not critically reviewed.

Sweden[5]

In Sweden an interesting experiment is going on with health education programmes in which the whole school environment is involved. Although these programmes are not necessarily organized by school health services they can play a role.

At Edsberg School in Sollentuna a health education model using group discussion with pupils and adults is currently being tried with an entire school year group. The theme of discussions is drugs, but other themes could be used. A group discussion model is used in which each class is split up into three smaller groups, with six to eight pupils in each group. In some cases an attempt has been made to keep friends together; in other cases new combinations of pupils have been tried. Two or three adult participants are assigned to each group of pupils, which means that about forty adults are involved in group discussions. Indirectly, all school personnel and pupils are involved to a varying degree by these group discussions and the processes they bring about. About half the adults taking part in the group discussions are teachers. The remainder are other school personnel — clerks, matrons, pupil welfare personnel from the municipal social services, recreation leaders from the youth centre and representatives of the church, the National Association of Tenants, clubs and, last but not least, parents.

Group discussions are held during school hours for eighty minutes a week. They have now been going on for three terms with the same group of pupils and the same adult participants.

This school has succeeded in creating the organizational conditions for regular group discussions for an entire form or year group at scheduled times, in small cohesive groups and with several adult participants in each group. The objective of group discussions was formulated as follows: to increase the ability of pupils to analyze their values, to reach decisions and heighten their self-confidence, and thus to better prepare them for the negative influences which they meet in everyday life, e.g., with regard to alcohol, drugs and tobacco. The belief is that with a small group of participants, all meeting over a lengthy period, there is some possibility of achieving a basic sense of security that helps each individual to examine the experiences affecting himself and others in his immediate surroundings. This applies not only to the pupils, but also in no small degree to adult participants in group discussions.

United States[6]

An interesting but not quite comparable experiment is going on in Hartford, Connecticut. The example is given because the underlying idea is relevant to purely preventive school health services. A six-year demonstration programme in a K-6 school in Hartford, Connecticut offers a model approach to demystifying health care and the acquisition of empowering health concepts and health care skills. At this school a comprehensive primary medical and dental service is available to all children. Technical, medical and dental services are provided in a strongly educational context. Each child is invited to be an active participant in his own care and to share in the care of peers, both in direct involvement at the point of intervention and at the level of supporting diagnostic strategies. Children assist the health professionals in self and peer care in a way which reveals the causal factors, nature and implication of a given pathology, and the rationale behind treatment options. Health education becomes synonymous with clinical care.

At the dental chair, for example, two children may accompany a third child receiving care and 'assist' the dentist in examining the mouth, identifying lesions, and preparing and administering treatment. Mystery is replaced by understanding; and the children sense the legitimacy and satisfaction in gaining control over an aspect of health which was previously frightening, painful and to be avoided. Teachers and parents are involved as resources and informed collaborators to ensure that the educational benefits are supported by classroom experiences and the home. The clinical learning/caring experience is an integral part of the educational policy of the school, not an appendage. The range of concepts and skills available through an in-school clinical service is, of course, not limited to pathological states. There are many opportunities for children to become involved in both health promoting and disease preventing activities. But it is clear that the active role of children in disease care gives highly focused hands-on experience which enjoys high credibility and provides concrete opportunities for observing the effects of causal factors and benefits of prevention and early treatment.

Switzerland[7]

In Geneva the Health Services for Young People are experimenting with health education programmes based on the provision of health information at different levels. The Health Education Section of the Health Services for Young People is responsible for giving precise directions concerning modes, organization, methodology and content of health education in different sectors of public schools. The different spheres of health promotion are trying to incorporate as many as possible the needs and expectations of the target public (children, adolescents, teachers and parents).

Health education takes the form of lessons, conferences, and debates which are attended by pupils, teachers and parents. These include:

Collective health education. Regular courses treat such topics as general health knowledge, prevention of addiction, sexuality, first aid, nutrition, hygiene and dental care. These courses are set up in collaboration with the teachers of primary and secondary schools. The main characteristics of these interventions are their systematic and obligatory nature and the involvement of parents. Before any action is undertaken, the service organizes a debate with parents, especially on the topics of addiction and sexuality. In the multidisciplinary approach to health promotion for young people, future teachers receive during their initial training a systematic health education course which is obligatory and which is organized by the Health Services for Young People. This course sensitizes them to the different health problems which confront young people. Appropriate audiovisual material is also prepared by the service.

Individual health education. This is done during each medical examination by doctors or nurses or the Health Services for Young People. The health education service is also available to parents, headteachers and teachers for any information they may require.

Possible Health Education Tasks of School Health Services

Our starting points for the formulation of possible roles in health education programmes are, first, the existing situation in which school health services work. Health education tasks demand only a reorientation of working methods and not a fundamental change in structure or means. A second starting point is the definition of school health services *sensu stricto*; this means school health services where the medical aspect is dominant, which is the most common situation. Taking into account the two main characteristics of school health services (medical dominance and sporadic contact), we see possible developments in health education as follows:

1　To provide basic information for school health education programmes:
— to signal existing medical problems;
— to inform and eventually train educators about medical problems.
The main objective is to base school health education programmes on actual needs of school children and on correct medical information.
2　To integrate health education elements in the periodic health examinations of pupils. The main objectives of these health educa-

tion activities are the stimulation of positive attitudes towards preventive health care and towards health care workers and the reinforcement of existing knowledge.

3   To provide the possibility of learning and training in such technical aspects of health education as first aid and dental care. The main objectives are to teach the techniques as such and to demystify technical medical aspects.

4   To promote and support the medical aspects of learning and training. The main objective is to provide optimal medical assistance for health education programmes.

Constraints and Obstacles to Health Education Activities

To return to the example of Belgium, we find that in the law on school health services there are several practical and financial problems which impede the reorientation of school health services:

1   Lack of time — legally imposed routine check-ups and administrative work mean that there is no time left for more intensive contact with pupils, parents and schools;

2   Lack of preventive orientation in training of health personnel in school health services;

3   The situation of the doctor within the school health services, with too large a proportion of part-time school doctors, resulting in organizational problems and a lack of motivation. The appointment of a full-time senior doctor is desirable. He should be responsible for coordination within the health team, for the revision of working methods, for contacts with outside organizations and for the organization of activities concerning health determining factors in and around the school;

4   The bodily and curative orientation of school doctors, because of their training and their normal activities outside the school health service;

5   A per capita payment for the examination of each child. Alternatively, a system in which the team were paid for the responsibility for the health of a certain school population would encourage more activities such as team discussions and more intensive and sustained contacts with schools, pupils and parents.

Conclusions

For the efficiency of school health education programmes the whole school environment must be involved; school health services have a role in these programmes. At present the discussion of health education is important because of the reorientation of school health services, and demands for integration of health education activities must be taken into account to ensure that these services can act as a useful component of school health education programmes.

Notes

1 *Evaluation of School Health Programmes*, Report of a WHO working group, Bucharest, 2–5 August 1977, p. 3.

2 WIERINGEN, J.C. VAN (1980) 'Jeugd gezondheidszorg als instrument van preventie', *T. Soc. Geneeskunde*, 58, pp. 52–5.

3 PARIJS, L.S. VAN (1980) 'Het medisch-educatief schoolonderzoek', *T. Soc. Genees-kurde*, 58, pp. 631–40.

4 PARIJS, L.S. VAN (1980) 'A new approach to health education in the school health service', unpublished paper.

5 FAXER, K. and SENNERFELT, P. (1980) Hopeful experiment. A report from two schools that are making use of the resources already existing in the school and its immediate vicinity', paper prepared for the WHO symposium on Constraints in Education for Health of Schoolchildren and Parents, Gent, 29 September–3 October 1980.

6 LEWIS, J. (1977) 'Towards comprehensive child health care: The school based delivery model', paper presented at the American Public Health Association, Washington, D.C., November 1977.

7 MOUNOUND, R.L. *et al.*, (1980) 'Le rôle des services de médecine scolaire dans l'éducation pour la santé des écoliers', paper prepared for the WHO Symposium on Constraints in the Education for Health of Schoolchildren and Parents, Gent, 29 September–3 October 1980.

From the Screening of Illnesses to Psycho-Social Support for Schoolchildren: A View from Finland

Matti Rimpelä

In Finland maternity and child health services were first developed by voluntary bodies, and since the 1940s by public administration. In preventive health the public health nurses had a key role, and improvements in the health of schoolchildren must be largely attributed to their work.

From the 1950s to the 1970s the prevalence of physical illnesses among schoolchildren decreased rapidly. Even so, most of the time of school nurses and doctors was taken up with screening physical symptoms and signs according to traditional routines. Awareness of the importance of early psycho-social problems became more widespread in the 1970s, the role of health education being especially emphasized. Nowadays we are searching for practical means of strengthening health promotion and providing psycho-social support as a key function of school health services.

An overall view of the present status of school health services in Finland, especially from the point of view of perceived health and psychosomatic symptoms, is set out below.

General Information

Finland, the easternmost of the Nordic countries, has a population of about 4.8 million and population density of 15.5 per square km. All persons over 15 are literate; school attendance is compulsory from 7 to 16 years of age.

Officials from ministries and national boards direct and supervise the local authorities. Health comes under the Ministry of Social Affairs and Health, and compulsory schooling under the Ministry of Education. The ministries supervise the national boards. The National Board of Health gives instructions about school health care, and the National Board of General Education about the goals and content of education. The country is divided into twelve provinces for the purposes of regional administration. The provincial authorities represent the state. The role of regional administration is increasing.

One important feature in Finland is the powerful tradition of local self-government, including the right of local authorities to levy income tax. The primary responsibility for providing health care and compulsory school education rests with local authorities, of which there are now about 460. Large communities have their own local boards. Small communities form federations of communities to run joint health care. The health board comprises a general department which looks after primary medical care, the local hospital and other forms of health care that together form the administrative organization known as the health centre.

In the early 1970s it was decided to put the main emphasis on preventive services and primary health care, and to create the necessary administrative and financial organization. The Primary Health Care Act was passed by Parliament in 1972. One major object was to provide comprehensive primary health care by integrating a number of services into a functional whole.

The Finnish health planning system is one of the rotating five-year plans which are reviewed annually. The national five-year plan is approved by the government, and the five-year plans of individual health centres have to be approved by the provincial administration acting on instructions from the National Board. One major difficulty is how to guide health policy without infringing the traditional autonomy of the municipalities (National Board of Health, 1978).

School Health Services

Finnish school health services began with the decision of the town of Tampere to hire a school doctor in 1900. In the 1920s and 1930s the number of school doctors increased rapidly; just before the Second World War there were about 300. There was a severe shortage of doctors in Finland until the late 1970s and their time was mainly taken up in screening physical illnesses and providing essential medical services. Finland has a well-established tradition of public health nurses working in local communes. An act creating health visitors came into force after the Second World War. By 1950 every local community had hired health visitors whose wide duties included responsibility for preventive health services in primary and secondary schools. In 1954 school doctor services covered about 99 per cent of schools and by 1969 97 per cent of local communes had organized dental health services for schoolchildren. According to the Primary Health Care Act of 1972, health centre staff provide all school health services. The National Board of Health issued new instructions regarding school health services in 1972 and a revised version in 1981. The aim of the latest directive is that health centres should hire at least one full-time health visitor per 800 pupils, and one full-time physician per 6000 pupils. Health centres in large communities have hired full-time public health nurses and pediatricians who are specialists in school health services. In smaller health centres school health personnel are only able to work part-time in the schools (National Board of Health, 1981).

One special problem in Finland is the division between mental and other primary health care. There is a separate mental health service with its own legislation. Specialized mental health services for children form part of this system. The health and social services are also run by two different administrative bodies. Personal social services are subject to a wide variety of regulations, implemented by different organizations. To make the picture more complex, schools have started to hire their own mental health and social workers. In 1979 about twenty communities had mental health workers who were specialists in schoolchildren's problems and who belonged to the school staff, not to the staff of a health centre or mental health services.

Health Situation

Mortality and Chronic Diseases

The health situation in Finland is characterized by low infant mortality and comparatively high adult morbidity and mortality. The infant mortality rate is one of the lowest in the world; in 1981 it was 6.5 per thousand. Since the late 1960s mortality has also decreased among middle-aged men and is now about 20 per cent lower than in 1969–70 (Central Statistical Office, 1982). Since the 1930s the health situation of women has been much better than that of men, judging by the incidence of serious diseases and mortality. In 1981 life expectancy at birth was 77.8 years for females and 69.5 for males. Mortality from all causes among 5–19-year-olds is no higher in Finland than in other Nordic countries. But a higher mortality rate among males is already apparent even in these age groups (see Table 1).

The most important obstacles to achieving a decrease in the mortality rate among schoolchildren are in the areas of accidents, injuries and suicides (See Table 2).

The hospital discharge register provides a picture of the health situation

Table 1. *Mortality from All Causes among 5–19-Year-Olds in Finland, 1970, 1975 and 1980*

| Age | Mortality per 10,000 | | | | | |
| | Females | | | Males | | |
	1970	1975	1980	1970	1975	1980
5–9	4	3	2	6	5	3
10–14	2	2	2	5	4	3
15–19	4	4	3	12	13	9

Matti Rimpelä (Finland)

Table 2. Causes of Death by Age and Sex in Finland, 1971–75 (percentages)

Cause of death	10–14-Year-Olds		15–19-Year-Olds	
	Females (266)	Males (455)	Females (496)	Males (1330)
Accidents	46	61	59	80
Malignant neoplasms	21	15	14	7
Congenital abnormalities	8	5	6	2
Diseases of the nervous system and sense organs	6	6	4	3
Diseases of the circulatory system	5	4	3	3
Diseases of the respiratory system	5	3	3	2
Others	9	6	11	3
Total	100	100	100	100

from the point of view of acute illnesses and accidents. In 1976 about 2.5 per cent of girls and 4.2 per cent of boys aged 12–14 years visited hospital. Between 5–14 per cent of schoolchildren suffer from some chronic disease according to various surveys and epidemiological investigations (Rimpelä *et al.*, 1983). In the 1970s the health situation improved among schoolchildren according to mortality statistics (see Table 1). However, the decline in mortality is smaller in this than in younger and older age groups. This unexpected phenomenon is mostly due to traffic accidents.

It has often been claimed in public discussions that the incidence of mental disturbances is rapidly increasing among youth. Mortality statistics and hospital discharge registers give only a very crude picture of the status of mental health. According to information from these sources, there are no clear trends in the incidence of serious mental illnesses in schoolchildren.

Two of the most common health problems found in epidemiological investigations are dental caries and allergic disorders. Dental health has improved rapidly among children and adolescents, although over 80 per cent of children still develop caries before the age of 16. According to various investigations, the prevalence of allergic disorders varies from 10 to 20 per cent. Some investigators have stated that the incidence of asthma and allergic disorders is increasing, but these statements have been challenged.

Perceived Health

It can be concluded on the basis of mortality statistics, hospital discharge registers and epidemiological investigations of chronic diseases that the health situation among schoolchildren is better than that among younger or older age groups. However, when perceived disability, especially psycho-somatic symptoms, are also taken into consideration the picture becomes more complex.

In Finland about 70 per cent of children of school-age reported a cough,

50 per cent a common cold and 5 per cent tonsilitis during the six months preceding a survey (Rimpelä, 1982). In this survey representing the whole population between the ages of 12 to 18 years irritability or fits of anger, headache and abdominal pains were the most common psychosomatic symptoms among 12-year-olds (see Table 3). About 10 per cent of girls and about 5 per cent of boys reported that they had experienced various kinds of psychosomatic symptoms often or continuously during the six months preceding the survey (Rimpelä *et al.*, 1982a).

Table 3.   *Prevalence of Most Common Psychosomatic Symptoms during the Six Months before the Survey among 12-Year-Olds by Sex (percentages)*

Symptoms sometimes or more often	Girls (506)	Boys (472)
Irritability or fits of anger	47	46
Headache	42	34
Abdominal pains	38	35
Excitement or nervosity	28	26
Difficulties in falling asleep, or awakening during nights	23	18

An alarming finding has been the widespread use of medicines. More than half the adolescents had used medicines during the month preceding the survey (see Table 4), 34 per cent for influenza or a common cold, 31 per cent for headache and 11 per cent for other aches and pains. Among girls who had passed the menarche, 10 per cent of the 14-year-olds and 17 per cent of the 16-year-olds had taken medicine for menstrual pains on several occasions during the preceding six months (Rimpelä *et al.*, 1982b).

Table 4.   *Use of Medicines during the Month Preceding the Survey by Age and Sex (percentages)*

Age (years)	Girls	Boys
12	59	47
14	65	59
16	64	53
18	73	45

Health Habits and Perceived Symptoms

In Finland adolescents usually start to use alcohol and tobacco between the ages of 13 and 16 (Ahlström, 1979; Rimpelä, 1979; see also Ahlström *et al.*, 1979). In this context the correlation of perceived health with health habits is more important than the incidence of smoking or use of alcohol. We found that the boys and girls who perceive their health as poor are likely to acquire

Table 5. Correlation for Psychosomatic Symptoms and Health Habits among 12-Year-Olds by Sex

Health habit	Girls (514)	Boys (483)
Smoking (daily)	.34***	.22***
Use of alcohol (often)	.25***	.30***
Time going to bed (irregular)	.23***	.24***
Use of traffic reflector (never)	.21***	.11*
Use of coffee (often)	.13**	.15***
Brushing one's teeth (seldom)	.13**	.08
Physical activity (slow)	−.03	.00

Notes: * $p < .04$
      ** $p < .01$
      ***$p < 0.001$

unhealthy habits (see Table 5). This correlation is especially applicable to those habits indicating irregularity of lifestyle in general, such as smoking, use of alcohol, irregular time of going to bed and poor dental hygiene (Rimpelä *et al.*, 1983).

Subjective assessment of poor health in general, psychosomatic symptoms and health-damaging habits seem to occur in some children even as young as 12 (see Rajala *et al.*, 1980; Honkala *et al.*, 1982, Laakso *et al.*, 1981).

Physical Maturation

Physical maturation is a very important phenomenon from the point of view of health education. It is well known that children mature at different rates, and reach the period of adolescence at different chronological ages. For instance, girls with adult female characteristics and boys whose puberty has not started can be seen together in a classroom of 13-year-olds. The rate and timing of physical changes at adolescence have significant concomitants in behaviour.

The rate of physical maturation can easily be measured by asking the age of the first period among girls and the age of the first ejaculation among boys. Our results show that there is significant correlation between early physical maturation and unhealthy habits among 12-year-old girls (see Table 6). The same relationship has also been found among boys (Rimpelä *et al.*, 1982c).

Another reason for stressing the importance of physical maturation is the timing of sex education. In Finland over half the girls reach sexual maturation at 12 or 13 and boys about one year later. No data are available about sexual activity among school children but the number of teenage pregnancies gives some information. The yearly incidence of estimated pregnancies (births and abortions) was 1/1000 among 14-year-olds, 16/1000

Table 6.   Health Habits among 12.6-Year-Old Girls by Age of First Menstrual Period
(percentages)

Health Habit	Age of First Menstruation		
	< 11 years	12 years	None yet
Daily smokers	4	2	0.3
Tried alcohol	27	19	16
Irregular physical activity	22	16	10
Irregular time of going to bed	21	17	10
Coffee more than two cups a day	15	9	8

among 15-year-olds, and 28/1000 among 16-year-olds in 1980–81. Teenage pregnancies have decreased by about 23 per cent since 1975, but more than three girls in every hundred will still become pregnant before their compulsory schooling has been completed (Kosunen and Rimpelä, 1983).

The Tradition of Screening

Instructions for school health services issued in 1972 by the National Board of Health concentrated on three areas of interest:

1   the health effects of the school environment;
2   personal health care of pupils; and
3   health education.

The objectives of health education were as follows:

to provide knowledge about matters concerning health and illness and to teach the required skills;
to create a positive attitude towards the topic being taught;
to maintain pupils' interest in the topic at all class levels by repeating and continuously bringing up new information; and
to get pupils to utilize the information and skills they have learned about health education and hence to adopt a healthy style of life.

The main function of school health services in the 1970s was the screening of physical illnesses. According to orders issued by the National Board of Health in 1972, height and weight was to be measured every year by the school health nurse. Special emphasis was put on the screening of albumin and glucose in the urine, anaemia, scoliosis and visual and hearing defects. Health examination took up most of the school doctor's time, with only a few minutes for each pupil in most schools.

In practice, school health personnel had only a limited amount of time for health education. The major responsibility for health education was placed on school subjects such as biology, civics, domestic economics, physical education, and hygiene. The amount of health education included in the university curriculum for different groups of teachers varies, and unfortunately is mostly very limited. It depends a lot on the teacher's own interests. Some consider that the themes of health education are important and have close cooperation with school health personnel, while others almost totally neglect their responsibilities as health educators.

New Instructions in 1981

During the late 1970s working groups set up by the National Boards of Health and Education reviewed the problems of school health services and health education and formulated proposals for instructions. In 1981 the National Board of Health issued orders for school health services from the point of view of organization, environmental questions and screening. New orders for mental health promotion and health education will be issued in the near future.

The goals of the new instructions are to direct a major part of available resources to mental health promotion, health education, and the care of chronic disorders and illnesses by economizing with a diminishing scale of screening routines. Height and weight will be measured every second year. The National Board of Health has recommended that only certain basic screening examinations be carried out, such as hearing and visual defects, anaemia of girls in the fifth and eight-grade and blood pressure in the first grade. According to the new instructions, yearly health examinations by the public health nurse and examinations by the school doctor of first, fifth and eight-grade pupils should stimulate discussion about individual problems and health education.

In practice, it seems to be very difficult to reduce physical screening examinations. For instance, professors in pediatrics are strongly against the recommendation to measure height and weight only every second year, considering that yearly measures should be continued. In Finland the prevention of cardiovascular diseases is one of the main tasks of health care. Many school doctors have suggested the screening of cardiovascular risk factors such as high blood pressure and cholesterol.

Summary and Conclusions

In Finland school health care covers the whole population of the age of compulsory education. We have well-educated school health personnel, but the tradition of screening physical defects and illnesses still dominates the practical work. There are no provisions for school health personnel to give health education teaching in the curriculum of primary and secondary schools.

Teachers have been given the major responsibility for health education, but only a few hours are reserved for general health education topics. The aim has been to integrate health education with many different subjects, but unfortunately, health education has only a limited role in the university curricula of teachers.

The time of school doctors is mostly spent in carrying out physical examinations. The public health nurse has yearly contacts with every pupil and more time for problem-oriented work. In the late 1970s the main emphasis was on health education concerning smoking, the use of alcohol and diet.

Data on the health situation of schoolchildren show that there are plenty of perceived health problems. A child's subjective assessment of his/her health as poor goes together with unhealthy habits and with problems in school work. Headaches and other functional symptoms indicate the aggregation of various problems in some children, even as young as 12 years.

Developmental age is as important a determinant of health problems as chronological age among schoolchildren. Family education should be strengthened, especially among early maturers, who also form an important target group for health education in respect of harmful habits.

Both the health education provided by teachers and the preventive health care provided by school health personnel have been based on the idea of dealing with the most common problems in each grade. Besides this approach, it can be seen that there is an urgent need for more individual and problem-oriented contacts with pupils. They need not only preventive screening and health education, but also help in caring for the symptoms and in solving daily problems. Pupils who have problems are well known by teachers and by school health personnel, and in many cases other members of their family also have contacts with the health and social services.

The main task of the future is the reorganization of school health care and daily activities, and also the development of qualifications of school health personnel in the direction of psycho-social support and the care of girls and boys who have problems and are seeking help. Another important goal must be the strengthening of the role of health education in the university curricula of teachers.

References

AHLSTRÖM, S. (1979) Trends in drinking habits among Finnish youth from the beginning of the 1960's to the late 1970's', *Reports from the Social Research Institute of Alcohol Studies No. 128*, Helsinki.

AHLSTRÖM, S. *et al.* (1979) 'The juvenile health, habit study — study design, methods and material' (English summary), *Kansanterveystieteen julkaisuja M48/79*, Tampere.

CENTRAL STATISTICAL OFFICE OF FINLAND (1982) *Statistical Yearbook of Finland 1981*, Helsinki.

HONKALA, E. *et al.* (1982) 'Consumption of sweet foods among adolescents in Finland', *Community Dent Oral Epidemiol*, 10, pp. 103–10.

KOSUNEN, E. and RIMPELÄ, M. (1983) 'Pregnancy among teenagers in Finland in

1965–81' (in Finnish), *Journal of the Finnish Medical Association* (submitted).

LAAKSO, L. *et al.* (1981) 'Relationship between physical activity and some other health habits among Finnish youth', in HAAG *et al.* (Eds) *Sporterziehung und Evaluation. Schriftenreihe des Bundesinstituts fur Sportwissenshaft*, Band 36, Verlag Karl Hofmann, Schondorf, pp. 76–81.

NATIONAL BOARD OF HEALTH (1978) *Primary Health Care in Finland*, Helsinki, p. 28.

NATIONAL BOARD OF HEALTH (1981) *Instructions about School Health Care* (in Finnish), Helsinki.

RAJALA, M. *et al.* (1980) 'Toothbrushing in relation to other health habits in Finland', *Community Dent Oral Epidemiol*, 8, pp. 391–5.

RIMPELÄ, A. (1982) 'Occurrence of respiratory diseases and symptoms among Finnish youth', *Acta Paediatr Scand*, Suppl. 297 (dissertation).

RIMPELÄ, M. (1980) 'Incidence of smoking among Finnish youth — a follow up study' (English summary), *Kansanterveystieteen julkaisuja M56/80*, Tampere, (dissertation).

RIMPELÄ, M. *et al.* (1982a) 'Perceived symptoms among 12–18-year old Finns' (English summary), *Journal of Social Medicine*, 19, pp. 219–33.

RIMPELÄ, M. *et al.* (1982b) 'Use of medicine and perceived health status among 12 to 18-year-olds in Finland' (English summary), *Yearbook of Health Education Research 1982*, National Board of Health, Finland, pp. 123–8.

RIMPELÄ, M. *et al.* (1982c) 'Sexual maturation and health habits' (English summary), *Yearbook of Health Education Research 1982*, National Board of Health, Finland, pp. 49–55.

RIMPELÄ, M. *et al.* (1983) 'Morbidity, mortality and perceived health of the Finnish youth' (in Finnish), *Publications of the National Board of Health, Health Education Original Reports*.

Oral and Dental Hygiene at School

Colette Menard

School Health Education

In France, although health education does not feature in official curricular instructions and handbooks as do history or physical education, it does appear at every level, as a development of many curricular matters, in 'awakening activities' (primary cycle) or in biology (secondary cycle). In the last four years, on behalf of the Health Ministry and with the cooperation of the National Education Ministry, the French Health Education Committee (FHEC) has launched important initiatives aimed at sensitizing children to their own health. Several programmes have been put into action.

1 Oral and dental hygiene for 5 to 6-year-old children (higher level classes of nursery schools),
2 Health education and life hygiene for 7 to 8-year-old children (elementary classes),
3 Tobacco education for 9 to 13-year-old young people (primary cycle),
4 Nutrition education for 6 to 12-year-old children (primary cycle).

A series of teaching materials has been prepared in keeping with the children's age, the type of teaching and the topic. Basically, it consists of:

materials for the teacher: 'the school teacher's document' which is a technical and pedagogic guide for planning activities by the teacher who is not yet trained in health education;
learning packs for the pupils.

The general principle is to give the child the opportunity of direct and active discovery, by experimentation, of the concepts which are to be explained.
    Set out below is one of these school health programmes — the oral and dental hygiene programme. The following points will be discussed:

1 oral and dental hygiene and epidemiological data;
2 general strategy for dental education programmes;
3 sensitization initiatives at the national level in higher level classes of nursery schools;
4 experimental study in a Regional Health Education Committee.

Oral and Dental Hygiene: A Public Health Problem

Almost all the population in France is affected either with dental caries or with diseases of the gums and teeth. Several epidemiological surveys, especially the national survey by the French Union for Oral and Dental Health (FUODH), involving 144,000 children, have shown the high frequency of dental diseases. For instance, whereas 61 per cent of 3-year-old children have no caries, only 2.35 per cent of 6–15-year-olds are in the same situation. Between ages 16 and 30 the percentage of teeth with caries or filled or missing is 43.5 and the average number per head doubles during this period. Most French and foreign studies show that from the age of 35 teeth loss because of periodontal disease increases steadily.

The cost of dental care is a very important part of the National Health Budget; in 1975 it represented 9 per cent of the total national health cost. The frequency of these oral and dental diseases could very often be reduced by the application of simple hygiene rules, efficient toothbrushing, healthy nutrition and periodic teeth examination. The socio-medical impact of these diseases should force the authorities to consider prevention as a priority and to improve information in support of it.

General Strategy for Dental Education Programmes

It would be useless to give young children information on good practices in oral and dental hygiene if their environment, more specifically their families, had not been sensitized to the subject. The communication strategy has been determined on the basis of the conclusions of a group of experts, and from the results of motivation studies. Two levels of objectives have been defined in parallel (see Figure 1).

First phase
sensitization of the child in his family context, through media, in order:
to change the fatalistic attitude of adults towards their teeth;
to provide the knowledge necessary for dental hygiene improvement;
to promote dialogue.

Second phase
in parallel, to teach good dental hygiene practice to children at school

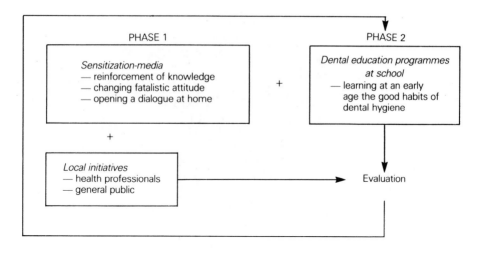

Figure 1. Strategy for Dental Education

Sensitization through the Media

In order to avoid giving offence and to get a good reception from adults and children, a distinctive communication style, using humour, has been chosen. The TV cartoon character 'Brossissimo' (Brushissimo) has been used for the promotion of two simple behaviours: efficient toothbrushing, and regular visits to the dentist. (In 1981 a new character was created, Archibald the Magidog, intended to promote, through several thematic episodes (dental hygiene being one of them), a global picture of health. This character has been used also in teaching material prepared for elementary classes in school.) The objective was to show that we can control the health of our teeth. The slogan 'our teeth are alive' illustrates this idea and opens up two clear directions: 'think about brushing your teeth' and 'get them examined regularly'. These spots are broadcast at regular intervals to ensure permanent sensitization (see Diagrams 1 and 2).

Local Initiatives

In parallel with the sensitization operations, information initiatives are undertaken for health professionals. These are relayed in the field through

Colette Menard (France)

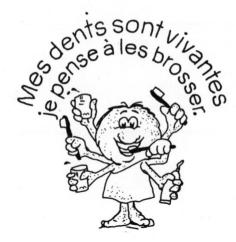

Diagram 1. *Brossissimo*

Diagram 2. *Archibald*

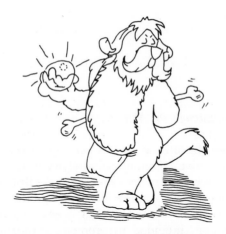

the distribution of materials edited for the committee campaigns (posters, brochures, stickers) by regional and local Health Education Committees, local committees of the National Association for Dental Health (FUODH), dentists, pharmacists, etc. In addition, debates, conferences, meetings, exhibitions are organized in the districts to increase the impact of the campaign.

National Sensitization Programmes in the Upper Classes of Nursery Schools

The education programme aims at informing 5–6-year-old children in upper nursery classes on dental hygiene. The theoretical aspect is concerned with acquisition of knowledge in this field. The practical aspect consists of helping children to integrate good dental behaviour into their everyday life. Teaching material has been prepared:

> for the teacher: a guide giving information on oral and dental hygiene, accompanied by twenty illustrated slides comparing teeth and plants as living organisms;
> for each pupil: an album with drawings to colour, a game of 'goose', a song, 'let's dance with Brushissimo', a toothbrush and a cup, a sticker 'my teeth are alive';
> for parents: a booklet on dental prevention and brushing technique;
> for classrooms: a poster 'my teeth are alive'.

This material is sent on demand, and the estimated take-up to February 1983 was 400,000 children involved in this campaign. It is intended that by 1984 more than 2 million children will have been sensitized to oral and dental hygiene.

National Evaluation of the Dental Education Programme

Every year a national evaluation is made through a questionnaire, in order to:

1 evaluate the reception of the campaign by teachers and parents;
2 test the effectiveness of the teaching material on children;
3 collect information on the children's reactions and their development.

1 *Reception of the campaign.* From the beginning this campaign has been very favourably received by teachers and parents. Thus, before it started 68 per cent of teachers and 71 per cent of parents thought that acquiring the skills of good oral and dental hygiene by young children depended on concerted action by parents and teachers. This opinion was subsequently strengthened by their experiences of the campaign when 72 per cent of teachers and 82 per cent of parents had a positive opinion of its educative effects.

2 *Content of the dental education programme at school.* If, at the beginning of the first campaign, some of the parents and teachers thought that the programme should be limited to the transmission of theoretical knowledge to children, by the end, their opinion was more in favour of a joint programme: transmission of theoretical knowledge *and* a real tooth-brushing apprenticeship.

3 *Use of the teaching material.* Slides are appreciated by teachers as a

means of lively transmission of basic knowledge about good dental hygiene. Children have a very positive reaction to them, showing their interest by asking many questions on the subject. The album 'Brushissimo' is appreciated because it is given personally and because it is funny. The teaching material is used in two-thirds of the classes, and some of the teachers claim to have used it several times.

As for dental hygiene practice, it seems that toothbrushing is established in a great number of schools and is carried out usually adjacent to the dining room or canteen. A very large majority of teachers (90 per cent) are of the view that children who have participated in the programme have benefitted.

If most of the teachers are enthusiastic and supportive, they also admit its limitations. To be really efficient, the experience must have the support and active participation of parents, so that the brushing practice and systematic examination of teeth by the dentist become a habit. In most cases, parents are informed of the programme undertaken in school. In the first survey: 13 per cent of parents said this experience had provided the opportunity for them to start the child's toothbrushing; 80 per cent estimated that it had helped them to intensify educative initiatives already undertaken at home; 70 per cent noticed a positive change in the child's attitude and desire to brush his teeth more frequently. Parallel with this behaviour evolution, there is significant progress in the sales of toothbrushes. The number of toothbrushes sold every year in France has increased by 45 per cent from 29 million to 42 million in 1981. During the last two years the most important progress concerns young children. Indeed, the sale of toothbrushes for children and juniors more than doubled, from 10 per cent to 25 per cent total toothbrush sales. The mean consumption of toothpaste also shows an increase from 95 gr per capita per annum in 1966 (i.e., one tube and a half) to 251 gr (i.e., a little more than four tubes) in 1981.

Experimental Study in a Regional Health Education Committee

The regional and local Health Education Committees have been closely associated with action at the national level and have themselves undertaken evaluations at the regional level.

For some of them the sensitization programme is an extension of work already undertaken. Thus, the RHEC of Beauvais has since 1972 given to 7–10-year-old children information on the benefits of dental hygiene. Because of this longstanding educational policy, the Oise district was chosen by the Health Ministry to try out an experimental programme of dental control at school, with the help of a specially equipped van. The programme had three phases:

sensitization and imparting information to the children;
teeth examination, on the spot;
treatment.

Although this experiment has been going on for five years, and made it possible to ascertain the impact of information on young children, until now no thorough study on this theme had been done because of lack of means. For that reason the RHEC, to encourage operational research in the field, decided to contribute technically and financially to the Beauvais Committee, to launch a small experimental study on information in relation to children's dental hygiene behaviour.

Aim of the Study

The aim was to determine the effect of information on young children's behaviour in oral and dental hygiene, by means of a long-term study. Bearing in mind the importance of the growth of teeth appearing at the age of 6, children from elementary classes (7–9-year-olds) were chosen.

Survey Methodology

The study was conducted over six months and was based on the principle of epidemiological studies, that is, on the comparison of two groups: a control group (receiving no information); an experimental group receiving information from the dentist, the teacher and several group leaders during the school year. To make comparisons possible, the two groups were drawn from similar populations consisting of one class from a city school (group I) and one from a rural school (group II). The evaluation was at two levels:

> *the epidemiological level* in order to: evaluate the dental state of each child (hygiene as well as dental care); determine if the child had been to the dentist during the last six months; verify the toothbrushing technique of each child. This part had been done by a dentist, during a visit of the 'detection van'.
> *the psycho-sociological level* in order to evaluate the opinion, knowledge and dental hygiene behaviour of each child. This was done through personal semi-directive interviews, by psychologists specially trained for that purpose.

The Survey

The pre-test. During October 1980 a pre-test was undertaken with the experimental group in order to have, even before the launching of the information campaign, an idea of the dental situation and knowledge level of the young children. The control group was not submitted to this first test so that no bias should be introduced in the data. The results of group I can be considered valid for group II, since the two samples were comparable.

Post-test.   This survey was undertaken in 1981 when the two groups were submitted to the same tests: epidemiological and psycho-sociological.

Information given by the health education group.   After the passage of the detection van, each pupil from the experimental group received a set of information on oral and dental hygiene by one or several group leaders from the health education service: slides, film projection (our teeth are alive), followed by a discussion and a toothbrushing demonstration with a model (big plastic jaws). In order to make his role more clear, the dentist provided information on the dental care he gives in his consulting room. He demonstrated once more the toothbrushing technique.

Information given by the teachers.   Each teacher gave information on his own initiative. The calendar of information sessions can be summarized as follows:

> *in the city school* (group I): four information sessions on oral and dental hygiene with texts and drawings;
> *in the rural school* (group II): teaching material (jaws and toothbrush) was exhibited in the classroom throughout the year. The information constituted the greatest part of the 'awakening activities'. The pupils built up a notebook with observations on the anatomy and physiology of teeth, on their role, on dental diseases and treatment. No regular sessions on toothbrushing were given because of lack of time and means.

It was then possible to determine without bias the incidence of information on the dental hygiene of children at home and on their dental state.

Evaluation

The survey determined that at the outset one-third of the children had never been to the dentist (20 per cent of the children in town and 47 per cent of the rural children). The preventive visit to the dentist was ignored or not well understood. Toothbrushing was related more to the idea of cleanliness than to real prevention. There was little knowledge about tooth disease. The information given during the school year had a significant influence on: opinion and knowledge expressed by the children on oral and dental hygiene, especially on prevention, disease detection by the dentist and toothbrushing efficiency; positive dental behaviour, with an increase in the frequency and regularity of toothbrushing. Seventy-five per cent of the children said that they brushed their teeth every day compared with 53 per cent before the experience. Among the former, 53 per cent brushed their teeth twice a day, 40 per cent three times a day, whereas at the beginning of the survey two-thirds of those who brushed their teeth did so only once a day.

On the dental aspect, the expectation has been realized of a real improvement in dental hygiene, particularly in the rural population where the imparting of information has been sustained, along with a moderate improvement in the care of teeth. On the other hand, the survey has underlined some difficulties specific to the rural environment: difficulty in reaching parents; maintenance of a number of false ideas: 'there is no need to take care of the milk teeth'; 'toothbrushing is useless'; dental care is considered costly and not a priority in the family budget; the difficulty of permanently providing dental care given the inaccessibility of dentists' consulting-rooms.

As the study reveals, information has a significant influence on children, who are interested by dental hygiene, but the information level must be sustained if it is to become really effective. It is desirable that dentists should be aware of this and be able to explain to parents the usefulness of regular dental care for their children. In the future it is also desirable that the detection of dental disease should be made more public, along with ensuring more permanent dental care at school.

Conclusion

Oral and dental hygiene have become a reality in school. The recent directives from the Health Ministry and National Education Ministry express a political will to develop more and more concerted action. School nurses and teachers will have the opportunity to follow training programmes by school health teams, alongside periods of instruction organized by the National Education Ministry. Furthermore, initiatives requested by education teams, parents and pupils will be undertaken, in the context of the three compulsory health examinations. Finally, the direction indicated must also lead to relevant research conducted in close cooperation with the Ministries of Education and Research and Technology. More and more initiatives are being taken to detect dental disease. Several French districts, following the lead of national associations such as FUODH, the Workers' Sickness Assurance, the National Federation of French Mutuals, have implemented dental prevention programmes of the 'detection' and 'information' kind. Thus whole school communities are concerned: children, teachers, parents, dentists, school health staff, and group leaders of regional and district Health Education Committees.

Health Education and the Environment in the Basic School Curriculum in Norway

Arne Hauknes

Historical Introduction

As in many other European countries, the intention of the first organized teaching in Norway was to prepare young people for confirmation in the church. This was tied to certain minimum requirements as regards knowledge of Christianity and morals. The term 'a sound mind in a sound body' was not entirely unknown, but the body should first of all be cultivated as a 'temple for the Lord'. Even if other subjects were introduced as time went on, only Christianity had its own special textbooks. From about 1850 religious authorities gave local school commissioners authority to extend the range of subjects; to the original subjects — reading, Christian knowledge, arithmetic, writing and music — were added natural science, geography and history.

In accordance with an Act Relating to Schools from 1860 natural science was included in the list of subjects. A curriculum published in 1877 stated, among other things, that natural science teaching will 'in connection with chosen texts from the reader, teach the children about the anatomy of the human body, its limbs, sense organs and its relation to nutrition, as well as the basic tenets of health education.' Further, 'it shall provide some basic knowledge of the methods used by Man to subdue natural forces for his own purposes.' Teaching was to be related to chosen texts in the reader, and the first reader became a subject for dispute because it included 'ungodly subjects'. Physical education (gymnastics), also mentioned in the Schools' Act of 1860, was for boys only, but the aim was, among other things, 'harmonious development of the body towards strength and fitness (health)'.

According to the 1889 Act Relating to Schools, subjects such as 'natural science, including the basic principles of health' should be given a special place in the timetable and have their own textbooks. However, teachers were poorly trained in these subjects. The first special textbook to include systematic information on anatomy, physiology and health education for the primary school was published in 1911. Very little happened in this area until a new Act imposing seven years of compulsory schooling throughout Norway was passed in 1936. This required a special curriculum expressing the objectives and minimum requirements for different subjects and topics.[1] The objectives for natural science teaching from the fourth grade in this Normal Curriculum include an item on health education: 'To give the pupils some knowledge of the human body, the basic principles of reproduction, and the most important rules of health, so that they are capable of protecting their health.'

The most important point in this new plan as far as health education is concerned was the introduction of a new subject, local studies. This included teaching in the mother tongue, natural science, geography, history, social studies and Christianity. The main purpose was to give children a proper basis for further education in these subjects, and to help them to understand their own role in the home, the school and the local community. Elements of health education form an important part of this subject. The choice of material includes important rules of health, information on substances damaging to health, transfer of infection through insects, first-aid in case of accidents, protection of nature, etc.

An important feature of this new curriculum was the introduction of Froebelian principles. Experiments and assignments which pupils solved for themselves, either in groups or with the teacher, were basic to teaching. The curriculum gives examples of several such assignments in health education, with guidelines on how to apply them in practice. The curriculum assumes that important health rules are discussed in every grade at school. In seventh grade the pupils have a special textbook on health education, with quite detailed information on anatomy and physiology. There are special syllabuses for topics relating to nutrition, to products/activities damaging to health, to the outdoor life, work and rest, clothes and the home, cleanliness and hygiene, etc. A special section deals with teaching concerned with the damaging effects of alcohol.

Health Education in the Present Curriculum

The 1969 Act Relating to the Basic School introduced nine years of compulsory schooling and a new Model Curriculum.[2] With certain revisions, this curriculum still applies today. Teaching in health education follows more or less the same lines as in the Normal Curriculum of 1939. But the extra two years' schooling gives more time for this topic.

In the Model Curriculum the basis for health education is found in 'local studies', taught in first to third grades. This is emphasized in the goals for the subject and guidelines for the teacher. Special topics are traffic behaviour, proper nutrition and dental care. Pupils also learn a little about how the body is made up and how it functions. The most important health rules such as cleanliness (hygiene), cleaning of teeth, etc. are followed up by the school and the home in partnership. The need for exercise, fresh air and sleep is also mentioned. More systematic natural science teaching starts in the fourth grade; the intention is to 'strengthen the pupils' ability and will to protect their own health and the health of others and to exploit natural resources in a proper and sensible manner.' In the fourth and fifth grades emphasis is laid on forming good health habits, particularly as regards food and drink, teeth and dental care, clothes and hygiene, fresh air, etc. In sixth grade pupils receive more detailed anatomy and physiology teaching.

Substances that are damaging to health, such as tobacco, alcohol and drugs, will have been mentioned already in the first to third grades, in connection with local studies. From fourth grade onwards these substances are discussed in more detail. The aim is to create a negative attitude towards them without making pupils want to experiment. In sixth grade pupils receive thorough instruction about these substances. Health topics are discussed in all grades when a natural situation for such discussion arises. In the last year of compulsory schooling (ninth grade) the curriculum includes a comprehensive health education course, with a special textbook. In all grades, from first grade onwards, it is considered important to develop a healthy and realistic attitude towards sex and reproduction, and sex changes in the body in relation to age.

Several health topics are compulsory in the course of a pupil's schooling. Special emphasis is placed on alcohol, drugs and tobacco. The curriculum gives guidelines for teaching these compulsory topics, and there is a whole series of textbooks for both pupils and teachers. Other compulsory health topics are nutrition, dental care, traffic sense, first-aid, and the environment and conservation.

There is also a special Act relating to the Health Service in Schools. This includes specific rules for routine health examinations, vaccinations and health guidance. In recent years the tendency has been to reduce this control programme and place greater emphasis on education and positive influence. It is usual for the school nurse to give guidance in health matters in all grades. Pupils can also visit the school's health centre for advice and assistance, and to get answers to specific questions. This perhaps applies particularly to girls, in connection with menstruation and contraception.

Health Education As an Integrated Element in an Environmental Project

The Model Curriculum gives both the school and individual teachers extensive opportunities to design and carry out teaching according to their own special syllabus or plan. Methods involving special topics and projects have been prominent, particularly in subjects belonging to the so-called

O-group (Orientation subjects), including natural science, health education, geography, and history with social education.

Even before the Model Curriculum was introduced the Institute of Educational Research at the University of Oslo had started planning a teaching project concerned with people and their environment. In recent years the project has been followed up and extended by the Basic School Council under the Ministry of Education, with comparable developments in other Scandinavian countries.

Reports on how man was destroying his environment (habitat), and on increasing pollution and its adverse effects on plant and animal life formed the background to this project. The question of conserving energy and other natural resources was also relevant. The Model Curriculum emphasizes the school's responsibility in promoting active protection of nature and the environment, and includes compulsory topics dealing with protection of health, nature and the environment as a whole. The main goals for environmental education are:

To provide:
1 insight into our natural, social and cultural environment,
2 an understanding of environmental problems and their be-haviural implications,
3 the motivation to work actively to solve these problems.

The Environmental Education Project includes a series of learning units for teachers, with specific examples to be used in teaching on the protection of nature and the environment. A major objective has been to clarify the relationship between goals, content, pupils' requirements and teaching activities. In a handbook for teachers working with this environmental project the authors point out:[3]

The general objectives place the main content of the unit in a general context.
The process objectives indicate the 'processes' or mental activities (for example, observing, experimenting, discussing) which, in our opinion should characterize instruction in the topic concerned.
The knowledge-related objectives point out those parts of the subject content to which it is important to direct attention.
The skills-related objectives show the skills which we wish to emphasize.
The attitude-related objectives indicate both attitudes, interests and values.

The project comprises four main areas divided into several extended topics:

1 knowledge and experience of the environment;
2 soil, water, air, noise, energy, problems of environmental pollution;
3 interrelationships in nature-eco-systems;

4 population, nutrition, health; the exploitation and distribution of natural resources.

Examples of learning units under the special health area (area 4) are:

A *Reproduction, puberty and population problems*
   1.08 The family
   1.10 Where do I come from?
   2.04 That's how I came into existence (conception-birth)
   4.07 What happens to my body?
   6.04 Are there too many of us?
B *Nutrition and utilization of resources*
   1.06 Our teeth
   2.09 Our packed lunch
   3.03 Food in other countries
   4.04 Take care of the sea
   4.05 What does hunger lead to?
   5.03 Food habits in developed countries
   6.05 Developing and developed countries
C *Alcohol, drugs, tobacco*
   4.08 You and I and both of us. Tobacco
   6.07 Do you want a smoke?
   6.08 Drugs
   6.09 Alcohol

Each learning unit was discussed by a group of specialists participating in the project and was tried out and evaluated in the schools before being presented to teachers as teaching material.

The learning units can be used in several ways in schools:

as a basis for teachers' education and advanced teacher training courses;
as references for information and ideas;
as resource books for a course on the protection of nature and the environment;
as a basis for discussion;
as a basis for teachers in groups preparing environmental education.

An Example of a Special Health Education Project: Smoking and Health

The Model Curriculum includes syllabuses and educational advice, and encourages the use of project methods in health education, especially for subjects dealing with the pupil's life and immediate environment.

Alcohol, drugs and tobacco make up one of the compulsory topics in the seventh to ninth grades and teachers have a distinct need for teaching syllabuses or plans and educational material. In 1978 the National Council on Smoking and Health started to prepare a special 'anti-smoking programme' for schools. The main objective was to develop teaching materials, try them out in practice, and assess the effects on pupils. This programme was based on earlier anti-smoking projects in schools. These had indicated that we should:

> focus more on the immediate rather than the long-term effects of smoking;
> give more attention to the social network surrounding and influencing the pupil's smoking behaviour;
> try to activate parents and persons in the immediate environment to participate in the educational programme.

From an extensive study of the smoking habits of Norwegian pupils aged 12 to 15[4] we knew that:

> more pupils were daily smokers when they came from homes where parents smoked and permitted their children to do so;
> the smoking habits of older siblings and of best friends were strong factors affecting the decision to be or not to be a smoker;
> the age of 13 is critical in this process. (At this age most pupils progress from the school for first to sixth grades to the school for seventh to ninth grades.

The First Stage: Anti-Smoking Programme Package

The first aim was to work out an anti-smoking 'package' for 12–14 year-olds in the basic school, using parental involvement as a key to influence. The reason for this strategy was the strong and independent effect of parents' restrictiveness on children's smoking habits. The 'package' comprised the following:

1 a folder for pupils, describing the immediate effects of smoking on the organism. This folder also discussed smoking as a form of self-pollution, and tobacco growing as a waste of agricultural resources;
2 a folder for parents, indicating that an anti-smoking campaign at school would probably have no effect without parents' active participation and support. They were also instructed in communicating with their children during the campaign in order to increase the effect on the children's attitudes and behaviour;
3 guidelines for teachers showing how to involve pupils in the campaign. It is well known that active participation, far more than passive listening, increases the probability that arguments will lead to change. One suggestion was to let pupils write an essay on

smoking and health. A general guide for the teachers describes their role in anti-smoking work in schools, and tells about available teaching material and where this can be obtained.

The Second Stage: Field Experiments

Two field experiments were carried out to test the effects of the material and the total school campaign. The first was worked out especially to test the short-term effect of the campaign on smoking behaviour of pupils.[5] Twenty-two schools in a rural district were divided into four groups.

1 In the first group of schools pupils were only given the folder constructed for use in the classroom. All other groups also received this folder, but other means were employed as well.
2 In the second group of schools pupils were actively involved by writing an essay on smoking and health.
3 In the third group pupils did not have to write an essay but parents were involved.
4 In the fourth group pupils and parents were actively involved.

In the fourth group the reduction in total cigarette consumption immediately after the campaign was trebled as compared with the first group. In the other two groups the reduction of cigarette consumption lay somewhere in between.

We concluded that it is possible to obtain a reduction, at least on a short-term basis, in the use of cigarettes among schoolchildren. The design of a campaign is of decisive importance, and even 'small' improvements can lead to an increased effect on children's smoking habits.

After the first field experiment, which also included interviews with parents and teachers, the material was changed and considerably 'improved'. The long-term effect of the revised material and campaign has been tested in a second field experiment conducted in an urban/rural area. It was concluded that the campaign had a certain long-term effect on those who smoked occasionally. In the first half-year after the campaign smoking rates decreased, although an increase had been expected. During the next six months the percentage of smokers increased at a lower rate than expected. The increase in this period was less than the increase which could be expected as pupils grew older. Therefore, after one year the 'net effect' of the campaign was still apparent.

Notes

1 *Normalplan for folkeskolen* (Normal Curriculum), Oslo, 1939.
2 *Mønsterplan for grunnskolen* (The Model Curriculum), Oslo, 1971.

3 NORWEGIAN ENVIRONMENTAL PROJECT (1975) *Teacher's Handbook*, Oslo, Institute of Educational Research.
4 AARØ, L.E. *et al.* (1981a) 'Smoking among Norwegian school children 1975–1980: 1. Extent of smoking in the age group 12–15 years, 1975, *Scandinavian Journal of Psychology*, 22, 3; AARØ, L.E. *et al.* (1981b) 'Smoking among Norwegian school children 1975–1980: 11. The influence of the social environment', *Scandinavian Journal of Psychology*, 22, 4.
5 AARØ, L.E., *et al.* (1982) 'Smoking among Norwegian school children 1975–1980: 111. The effect of anti-smoking campaigns', *Scandinavian Journal of Psychology*, 23.
6 BEWLEY, B.R. *et al.* (1976) *Smoking by Children in Great Britain. A Review of Literature*, London, Social Science Research Council and Medical Research Council.

The Multicultural Background to Health Education

Mary Holmes

The Health Education Council for England and Wales sponsored a small feasibility study to identify ways in which ordinary teachers in English schools might be helped to provide health education acceptable to the broad range of ethnic groups now in our multicultural society. It seemed sensible to look at the task in terms of general cultural diversity rather than to focus, yet again, on minority groups — hence the title.

There are some who say that this is a small problem and that in health education there is much else to do. It may appear a small problem in rural areas but in a number of inner cities up to 40 per cent, and in some schools up to 90 per cent, of the population may be black. It is probable that some minority groups have a greater need for health education than the white majority. Statistical evidence on the health of immigrants is difficult to come by and to interpret, but the 1980 Black Report, *Inequalities in Health*, states, 'what little evidence that has been accumulated ... does suggest that the children of immigrants do suffer from certain specific health disabilities related to cultural factors such as diet or to their lack of natural immunity to certain infectious diseases. Studies ... have pointed to the possibility of higher than average morbidity associated with maternal deprivation.'[1]

After discussing the evidence for inequality in health service availability and use, which shows the working classes at a considerable disadvantage, the Report says:

> it is likely that similar conclusions would follow from a considera-
> tion of race and ethnicity ... Coombe has referred to hesitation in
> seeking antenatal care among immigrants and their difficulty in
> securing adequate dietary information. There is evidence of some
> lack of appreciation among health service staff of the special needs of
> some immigrant groups as well as a clear lack of adequate facilities
> in some areas in which they have been obliged to congregate.

Alix Henley's work[2] makes an important contribution towards a solution of this problem within the health service but schools also have a part to play, not only in areas with a high immigrant population. We live in a multiethnic society wherever we may teach. It was multiethnic long before the post-war boom in immigration to the United Kingdom, and for generations the white population has been multicultural in terms of social class factors and religious background. We could take advantage of this diversity and seek from it enrichment of our curriculum. In April 1980 Baroness Young, then Minister of Education, reiterated this view:

> It is just as important in schools where there are no ethnic minority pupils for the teaching there to refer to the different cultures now present in Britain, as it is for the teaching in schools in the inner areas of cities like Birmingham and London. It is a question of developing a curriculum which draws positive advantage from the different cultures.

All teachers need to be aware of this and to educate children, even in areas where multiethnicity is not visually apparent, to be sensitive to this diversity.

Health Education in a Multicultural Context

It is now generally recognized that behaviour conducive to health depends on a positive self-image. 'Self-image' is probably one of the most important concepts in health education today. It is also one that has been considered in some depth by those who are concerned about minority groups. We need to ask if health education materials contribute to the development of a positive self-image for all minority groups and social classes.

The giving of specific information is also part of health education. Information about our health and social services and *how to use them* is badly needed by immigrants and slow learners at the school stage and beyond. Are there adequate materials for use in schools on the use of services and on health and safety measures at work?

Health education is by its nature concerned with sensitive issues. If we as teachers 'offend' either by insensitive comment or inappropriate visual materials, we are wasting our time — the message will be rejected. We are often unaware of the strong cultural and sometimes irrational basis for our own habits. How many of us could knowingly eat dogmeat? What, after all, is the 'health' basis for our very strong desire for privacy and indoor WCs? Feelings about food, personal behaviour, hygiene and marriage customs are always strongly held and may have considerable bearing on health behaviour.

How, then, can we help ordinary teachers to be more sensitive to the cultural background of the children they teach? There are three main areas of concern:

1 illustrations;
2 specific information;
3 sensitive issues;

and the last is by far the most difficult to deal with.

Strategy

It was distressing to find that, as in the population at large, there are some teachers who feel that no special consideration should be given to minority groups. It is also important to recognize that sensitive material concerned with cultural differences may be open to misuse. Furthermore, although some ethnic minorities and other social groups do strive to maintain and to protect their own cultures, many do not want to be singled out. A number of people with whom this was discussed felt that as often as possible issues to be considered, e.g., diet, should be seen as *cultural enrichment* rather than as problem areas. After all, foreign travel is seen in this light. Why should not the varied groups within our own country be seen to contribute similarly?

In some of the schools visited social evenings were organized by parent-teacher groups with this as an objective, but relatively few schools seemed to incorporate such diversity into the curriculum for all pupils. A review of examination syllabuses might throw some light on this situation.

What Might Then Be Done?

The illustrations for all health education materials should indicate that our society is multiethnic and multicultural. It is not easy to get the balance right. One headmistress of an infant's school said that she had complaints from parents if the children's work on the classroom walls became too 'Chinese' or too 'Asian'. She checked weekly to see that a balance was kept. It is, of course, a measure of her success in helping children to accept their own identity that they could, and did, illustrate themselves as they were — black, brown, white or yellow. Many black children in schools still consistently draw themselves as white skinned.

Health information materials could be written in such a way that they could be used in language courses or for slow learners in science, social studies and 'leavers' courses looking towards adult life. *Speak for Yourself*, a BBC programme, has provided a useful example.

There is much evidence to indicate that further attention should be paid to the use of health and social services in schools where everyone can be reached. There is a good deal of material already available at community relations centres, various LEA multi-ethnic and language centres and in health education projects. Henley makes an important contribution in her book, *Asian Patients.*[3] A primary school version, *People Who Help Us*, would be a useful addition.

The TUC has recently drawn attention to the need to make sure that *health and safety measures* are understood. School leavers and careers courses could be provided with materials on this with a multiethnic bias, again in very simple and direct language.

There is ample evidence, e.g., in Royal Society of Health journals, that, with changes in lifestyle, *building materials and heating methods*, many houses suffer badly today from condensation. How to avoid this is not generally understood, least of all perhaps by people from hot countries whose main concern in England is to keep their houses warm. Bad ventilation and high humidity may well lead to respiratory ailments and cross-infection. Drawn curtains and being kept indoors may prevent what little sun we have from reaching children, who need sunlight on their skins for the production of vitamin D. The HEC already has an interesting leaflet on 'Safety in Your House'. 'Ventilation in your House' might follow.

Discussion of WCs and their use is to some extent taboo among most groups in our society. Their placing and maintenance are often causes of complaint by Environmental Health Officers. Many immigrants do not understand our *housing regulations* and their scientific basis. A leaflet could examine these issues in such a way that the subject could be introduced into science or social studies to give immediate and relevant understanding of domestic problems (replacing some of those boring lessons on 'the sewage works' that form parts of some biology courses!). Leaflets on housing regulations for use in schools might be prepared by Environmental Health Officers with help from 'English as a second language' experts. This might also provide an opportunity, through the children of the family, to prepare the women of the household for the statutory inspection of kitchens and WCs by male officers, which many Asian women find both frightening and offensive.

With regard to *food*, so much attention has already been paid to it locally and there is so much material already available that perhaps a home economist should be asked to collect and review material for the purpose of producing something nationally at both primary and secondary levels which emphasizes cultural enrichment as well as health needs, e.g., vitamin D, nutritional value and cost of vegetarian meals. Such a booklet should appeal to the ordinary child or young person and to parents and other adults, and might be called 'Why not try this?' It should also include geographical information about the origins of food and recipes to reinforce children's knowledge of their homelands. A secondary school version should not only make a contribution to examination courses but also provide ideas for bachelor cooking courses so that boys are not left out. A review of the multicultural content of food and nutrition examinations might be carried out at the same time. Food hygiene should be included. Asians often find our methods of washing up unacceptable; and not all teachers may know why Asians do not use their left hands for mixing and eating.

Biologists should also know about attitudes to food and hygiene. It is their job to make sure the basic scientific reasons for various practices are understood. They also need to know a little about health problems of immigrants and are likely to be asked to teach human physiology, including reproduction. They need to be aware of varying attitudes to discussion of the human body and to sex education. Notes on the teaching of biology in multi-ethnic situations might alert them to sensitivities and offer a booklist for further reading. Even ordinary teaching about the human body and its functions to boys and girls together, particularly by a male teacher, may be deeply offensive to some Asians. We may not be able to avoid this, but at least we should be aware of children's feelings. We should perhaps also reconsider the use of films in this context — particularly of child birth. Why do we expect teenage children to watch on film a traumatic process that only those entering the medical profession ever need watch from that view point?

Sensitive Issues

For teachers who are already interested in finding out about religious and cultural differences there is no shortage of books and lists of materials. The difficulty is to reach the ordinary teacher who perhaps no longer sees coloured pupils as very different from the rest, and does not question the effect of strongly held religious beliefs among the white population any more than the black on what they see as essential education about nutrition, eating habits, hygiene and reproduction. For them *brief notes* need to be included with other health education materials, with suggested further reading. *Starting School*, by Brian Jackson would be enjoyed by both primary school teachers and those teaching childcare in multi-ethnic areas.[4] *Asian Patients* by Alix Henley should be read by anyone teaching human biology and sex education.[5] Material from this could be easily adapted for school use, possibly in leaflet form.

Sex Education

Sex education is once again being singled out for particular attention in schools and it would be no quick or easy matter to provide adequate guidance for multi-ethnic situations, though many schools are attempting it with great sensitivity. Teachers do need help, but this task should not be undertaken without further consultation. In the meantime, Dr Elphis Christopher, in *Sexuality, Birth Control in Social and Community Work*, has a chapter on 'The influence of religion and culture', which many teachers would find useful.[6] This might be adapted and reprinted for school use. She is also preparing a book on *Sex Education in Schools*. In the meantime, a conference on the life cycle would be helpful. At one college it was suggested that 'what is needed, is not necessarily additions to the list of proper concerns of the health education teacher, but a better informed, multi-cultural approach to this content. This might be best undertaken by a systematic consideration of key issues faced by human beings as they move through the common path of physical, psychological, social and spiritual development from prebirth to death.'

Child Care Courses

Child care courses could provide an easy market for a series of leaflets in which cultural diversity could be seen as enrichment. There is already collected material, and the need is great not only in terms of children's acceptance of their own identity but also because of the lack of knowledge among young, white, middle-class home economics teachers who are often given these courses to teach. Such pamphlets once prepared could also be used in primary school and social studies courses. Titles might include:

The first few weeks, religious and other customs affecting the new baby, clothing, bathing, feeding, etc.
Naming the baby (see BBC *Speak for Yourself*) and Alix Henley's *Asian Patients*
Festivals and celebrations, including weddings
Party foods
Play and toys
Children's stories
Songs and lullabies
Family structures, courtship, sex roles
Sex education and family planning
Good manners, introducing ideas on discipline, control of young children and ways to speak to people acceptable in different societies, and what is usually expected in our own.

Summary

All these suggestions should be seen primarily as cultural enrichment through diversity. The medical profession must of course be equipped to deal with specific health problems, but within the schools and the community, people, particularly children, who have come to live in this land must be accepted, their contributions seen as enrichment, and welcomed.

Notes

1 BLACK, D. (1980) *Inequalities in Health*, (The Black Report), London, DHSS.
2 HENLEY, A. (1979) *Asian Patients in Hospital and at Home*, London, King Edward's Hospital Fund for London.
3 *Ibid.*
4 JACKSON, B. (1979) *Starting School*, London, Croom Helm.
5 HENLEY (1979), *op. cit.*
6 CHRISTOPHER, E. (1980) *Sexuality and Birth Control in Social and Community Work*, London, Temple Smith.

Using Science and Health Teaching to Enable the Disabled

Herbert D. Thier

In the United States health education is a minor part of the educational experience of most students. Especially at the elementary and early secondary school level, health education, if it takes place at all, consists of reading out of a book about body systems, hygiene and diseases. Even where health is mandated by state or local education codes, the usual program consists of reading the health book once a week, if as often as that. Certain schools and school systems (especially where there is a professional health educator on the staff) have much more extensive instructional programs, but these are the exception rather than the rule. At the upper elementary and early secondary school, topics such as sex education, drugs, alcohol and smoking are frequently taught as special programs (sometimes by parents or other outsiders) and this may be the only health education to which the student is exposed.

With the exception of the Health Activities Project (1980), there are few health education materials available that involve students with their own health and safety through hands-on discovery activities. This kind of program encourages students to investigate their own capacities and therefore learn first-hand how their body functions. Through this kind of health education students become aware of the control they have over their own health and safety and how both can be improved. Recent research (Voss, 1983; Bredderman, 1982) at the elementary school level has shown that students exposed to such hands-on discovery-oriented programs in science had higher achievement scores than comparable students exposed to more traditional textbook-oriented science programs. Science experiences are valuable and important in the development of all learners. As will be shown in this chapter, these experiences are essential if physically disabled individuals are to achieve their academic and social potential.

The overall purpose of this chapter is to describe and explain the unique and essential role early and continued science experiences can play in enabling disabled individuals to develop their potential to the fullest. The ideas expressed are based on the experiences of the author and his colleagues in developing such science experiences for physically disabled learners and their peers. Some of the extremely important health related values of such instruction for the disabled will be highlighted. The assumption is that the development and/or adaptation of hands-on, experience-based, science related health activities, like the Health Activities Project (HAP), for disabled individuals would further accomplish these values in addition to providing disabled learners with the educational benefits described above of health programs like HAP. It is necessary to first look briefly at the nature of science teaching and at the nature of disabled individuals. Then it will be shown how science experiences can be used to accomplish a wide variety of specific objectives, while enriching and enlarging upon the educational and life experiences of disabled individuals.

Nature of Science Teaching

Education is the learning of facts and how to use them as part of decision-making about problems and issues of concern and importance to individuals and the society in which they live. If all that education does is provide facts, the result is human encyclopedias. On the other hand, if education tried to teach decision-making without a factual reference frame, chaos would soon set in.

At a conference on the American high school in 1982 Gus Tyler described education succinctly as a combination of rote and reason (Tyler, 1982). Rather than waste time arguing whether rote or reason is more important, our responsibility as educators is to find ways to effectively and efficiently blend rote and reason to bring about quality education for all. Learning to read, write, and compute requires considerable rote learning, especially in the elementary and early secondary school. Each subject can provide many opportunities for strengthening the reasoning side of education, but usually the only reasoning is related to how effectively one has mastered the rote side of education. For example, if one does not know the times tables, word problems involving multiplication are very difficult, time consuming, and virtually impossible to handle.

Science, with its emphasis on evidence and use of mathematics and natural language, can provide unique opportunities for all students to use and develop their reasoning abilities. Whether or not this takes place is determined by the kind of science taught. Biology at any level, for example, can be another foreign language concentrating on the learning of new words to name and describe organisms and processes. It can also be an introduction to the wonders of life and all of the opportunities for analysis, synthesis, and greater understanding which become available with its study. Facts are needed, but the quality of the science program is determined by the context in which the facts are learned. The learner can be considered an empty vessel to be filled with certain facts each class period or week and then evaluated by how many facts the vessel is able to accurately pour out of its spout. This type of science program is focusing only on rote and is a poor excuse for science teaching. On the other hand, if each science class is another disconnected 'gee whiz!!', 'magic-like' experience provided at the end of the day 'because the students are too tired to learn anyway', then at best you have experience for the sake of experience. That also does not come close to the possible educational potential of the science program.

Quality science teaching at any level is 'experience-based'. The evidence collected by the learner is combined with the factual and procedural input provided by the teacher and other sources in order to evolve in the learner the knowledge, confidence, and interest necessary for effective decision-making. Therefore, the competent science teacher blends direct and indirect experience with the necessary factual and procedural input in order to accomplish what we will refer to as *experience as the basis for guided learning*. Such an approach to science teaching includes the 'rote', but certainly emphasizes the 'reasoning' aspect of education. Especially for the disabled learner, science provides many opportunities for necessary related learning experiences in fields such as mathematics, language, and everyday application skills.

Nature of the Disabled Learner

The term 'handicapped' traditionally was often used to categorize individuals in order to describe what they could not do and how we, the non-handicapped, had to take care of them. The term comes from the old English and evolved to describe the begger 'cap in hand' asking for alms. Too often our approach in education has been similar. We tested so-called 'handicapped' individuals, determined what they could *not* do, then described an educational program for them that emphasized care and dependence. Done many times for what were thought to be the best of reasons, such approaches were and are unfair to both the individual and society. Individuals are discouraged from achieving their potential for independence. This commits society to implied acceptance of a life-long period of costly care for and dependence by the individual. Essentially, such programs 'cap the handicapped' by determining early what they cannot do and then adjusting both their educational programs and their aspirations to these limitations. We have had extensive experience working with seriously disabled youth ranging from the congenitally blind to the severely cerebral palsied (no verbal speech). Our experience indicates that for all disabled youth there is significant potential and capability for learning. Needed is an instructional system designed to maximize their capabilities and minimize their disabilities. Disabled individuals tend to lack some of the experiences of their non-disabled peers. They tend to be highly motivated to learn, especially when you are able to design an instructional experience so that they can really take part in it. Disabled individuals tend to lack some of the experiences of their non-disabled peers. They tend to be highly motivated to learn, especially when you are able to design an instructional experience so that they can really take part in it. Disabled individuals then explore and extend their own limits rather than having outsiders arbitrarily set limits for them based on what the outsider believes a person with that disability can do.

Science Experience and the Physically Disabled Individual

The educational emphasis necessary for the disabled is one of 'Enabling the disabled rather than capping the handicapped'. Research studies to determine what disabled individuals cannot do are unnecessary. We need first to identify the critical information, ideas, and issues necessary to understanding a topic. We can then work on developing and/or adapting and testing an instructional system that enables disabled individuals to gain that understanding in a context that contributes to their self-confidence and self-image. School can only be an introduction to learning if we consider learning to be a life-long endeavor. Therefore, for disabled individuals, just like their non-disabled peers, it is necessary to transmit and develop the information and understanding needed by individuals to become independent, contributing members of society. In addition, and more important, it is necessary to help individuals, disabled or not, to *learn how to learn*. Then, whether it be in the world of work or as participating citizens in our democracy, individuals will be able to adapt to changes, process and analyze new information, and make intelligent decisions based on the evidence. Especially in relation to making intelligent decisions about their own health and the life-long care and conditioning of their bodies, all individuals, disabled or not, need to learn how to learn from their everyday experiences. Society is becoming more dependent on science and technology and citizens are expected to make a wide variety of science and technology-based decisions. Therefore, science and related fields have become extremely important in the educational experience of all learners. For disabled learners, science instruction starting at an early age and continuing throughout their school career takes on added importance for the following reasons:

1   Science emphasizes hands-on experience and exploration of the environment, both physical and biological. It can help to fill some of the experiental gaps in the background of many physically disabled individuals. Whether these gaps have evolved because of extensive hospital stays, overprotectiveness of schools and parents, or a variety of other reasons, these experiences are essential in developing knowledge and understanding of one's environment and one's

personal relationship to it. Such understanding is extremely important in helping to develop the individual's independence and
positive self-image.

2   Recent scientific and technological advances have provided tools
(computers, talking calculators, control systems, versabraille hook-
ups to computers, TTY telephone systems, etc.) which can help to
mitigate the limitations imposed by disability. This can enable
disabled individuals to be independent contributing members of
society. In order to effectively use these technological devices,
disabled individuals need first to know about them. Also helpful is a
variety of experiences exploring variables, using equipment and
materials, and generally getting over fear and apprehension regarding machines and related devices. Many of these technological
devices involve organizing and inputting information. Science
instruction with its emphasis on making observations, collecting
and organizing evidence, and coming to conclusions can be helpful
in developing the individual's psychological and manipulative readiness for using technological devices.

3   Job opportunities in the future will require greater knowledge and
understanding of technological devices and how they work. The
computer will be important in many jobs. Because of technological
advances in alternate ways for individuals to use computers, many
of these jobs are available even to the seriously disabled if they have
the necessary background and training and, perhaps more important, self-confidence. As described above, early experience-based
science education can help disabled individuals to develop the skills
and attitudes necessary to effectively take their place in the world of
work as independent contributing members of society.

Designing and implementing a science program is a complex and
demanding task. Instructional experiences and materials need to be selected,
the approach to instruction needs to be decided and the involvement of
learners needs to be planned effectively. This is true whether or not the
group includes physically and/or learning disabled individuals. Since mainstreaming is to a great extent the philosophy of education in the United
States, and science or health program, especially at the elementary and early
secondary level, is likely to include one or more learning and/or physically
disabled individuals.

In our work over the past thirteen years, designing materials and
instructional approaches for physically and learning disabled individuals of
all ages, two consistent outcomes have emerged. First, irrespective of how
disabled the individual or group may be, there is a way to help them have
interesting and effective experiences that lead to understanding. Secondly,
any time we have come up with a modification that has enabled disabled
learners to experience and understand some aspect of science more effective-

ly, that adaptation has proved to be an outstanding science experience for all learners, especially the non-disabled. Therefore, the principles and approaches described below to help meet the specific and unique needs of disabled learners are really principles and approaches for effective science teaching for *all* learners.

In summary, physically disabled individuals have deficiencies and cannot perform certain functions in the same way as the non-disabled, or in some cases cannot perform them at all. A great deal of educational planning and programming for the disabled has focused on these deficiencies and what individuals could not do rather than the adaptive approaches to meet the individual's needs. Significant legal and policy changes in the United States have set the stage for a more enlightened view of the physically disabled and their educational needs. Technological and scientific advances, especially in alternative modes of exploring and expressing ideas brought about by advances in computers and related fields, have gone a long way towards minimizing the individual's disability and maximizing capabilities. Science education which emphasizes *experience as the basis for guided learning* can play a unique role in providing young physically disabled individuals with information, understanding, and experience. This can help them become capable of, and have self-confidence to benefit from, opportunities available through technology.

Selecting Instructional Experiences and Materials for Disabled Learners and Their Non-Disabled Peers

The nature and complexity of science or health is such that no course or total school program can hope to cover all aspects. Choices need to be made which determine the nature and impact of the learner's experiences. Many elementary and junior high school textbook series survey as many aspects of science or health as possible and so provide interesting facts and information about a great many topics. They even highlight the variety of topics covered in scope and sequence charts. Often such a choice leads to a 'reading about science or health' program, with the textbook becoming the core of the program and actual science or health experiences supplementary or optional. Contrast this with a program like the Science Curriculum Improvement Study (SCIIS) (Thier *et al.*, 1978) at the elementary level or the Health Activities Project (1980) at the upper elementary and early secondary level. Here a hands-on approach is used to get across a selected set of content and process objectives. The intent is to develop an understanding of the nature of science or health or parts of them as a field of inquiry. The emphasis is on the learner actively participating in the learning experience, collecting evidence, using the evidence to make decisions, and then using those decisions to organize ways to collect new evidence. Far fewer topics can be introduced and fewer facts are learned; the emphasis instead is on scientific thinking. The 'reason' rather than the 'rote' side of education, as described by Mr Tyler, is emphasized. We have found this kind of science, with its emphasis on *experience as the basis for guided learning*, to be so beneficial for disabled learners and their non-disabled peers.

Determining the Approach to Instruction for Physically Disabled Learners and Their Non-Disabled Peers

Once the commitment to use experience-based multisensory science or health materials has been made, some of the approaches to instruction are already determined. For example, we can expect that learners will be spending much of their time exploring materials and gathering evidence rather than reading in a science or health textbook. Experience for the sake of experience with no other input is, however, a very inefficient way to foster real learning. What is needed are effective, challenging materials for individuals to explore, combined with carefully planned interventions by the teacher or other instructional leader. Instructions, diagrams, and work or record sheets can serve some of this purpose of organizing and directing instructional experiences. None of these approaches currently can provide the reflective interaction and personal understanding provided by the knowledgeable, interested instructional leader. Continuing advances in computer-assisted and other automated approaches to instruction can provide some of this guidance and direction for hands-on experiences without the use of the human instructor. The value for all learners, especially the disabled of human interaction with a knowledgeable leader is essential. Disabled or any other learners may have problems working with any automated system of instruction and need help. More important, especially for the disabled, is the fact that no machine can judge the temperament, emotions or unspoken desires of the learner. The teacher, based on continuing interaction with the individuals, can know when to probe further, when to accept an answer even if it is not perfect, and even more important, when to provide learners with additional time to explore further on their own or to just 'mess around with materials' (Hawkins, 1965) before introducing a new concept or asking for the kind of thinking that brings about conclusions and decision-making. Especially for physically disabled learners, who may be sensorially and/or experientially deprived, this kind of time for self-directed or autonomous learning is very important. Karplus (1981) has contrasted these two aspects of the instructional approach as 'autonomy' and 'input'. Effective instruction includes carefully planned opportunities for both autonomy and input on the part of the learner. However, autonomy does not mean total freedom any more than input refers to rigidity. Critical to quality instruction is the differing roles played by the teacher during periods of autonomy and input for the learner. For example, the kind and quantity of instructional materials, printed or other instructions, and the overall learning and emotional environment all contribute directly to the value and effectiveness of autonomous activity by the learner. The teacher's role is very important in selecting and sequencing opportunities for learning in relation to the overall objectives for the program and the prior experience and demonstrated capabilities of the individual learner. Learners are primarily involved in independent activity working on their own or in collaboration with peers. The teacher should be available as an intelligent observer ready to step in and help individuals or groups. The teacher should not break in so often that the learner's train of thought is interrupted and opportunities to benefit from successes and failures are taken away. When teachers should or should not become involved is a matter of judgment related to the materials being explored and the learners doing the exploring. Instructors who are constantly breaking in to be helpful need to reassess their role.

The situation is more complex with seriously physically disabled learners. Some will need the help of an instructor, attendant, or peer very often during many learning experiences if they are to be beneficial. Careful selection of activities and adaptation of materials and devices can help, but for some learners significant assistant will be required. Even in extreme cases real autonomy for involved learners can be provided with careful planning. For example, a teacher was working with a severely cerebral palsied girl on a life science activity investigating variables in the growth of root vegetables. Students were instructed to plant one whole root vegetable in vermiculite, right side up, and then to plant other root vegetables or parts of root vegetables upside down, sideways, etc. to see if they would grow and in what direction. With minimal instructions the activity provided great autonomy for participants. The girl with cerebral palsy could plant no root vegetables since she had very limited controlled use of her hands. The teacher (a paraprofessional who knew her well) explained the possibilities and then let the student gesture and otherwise communicate to explain which vegetables she wanted to plant, whether she wanted to plant all or part of each and in which direction. The teacher then planted all of the vegetables for her and helped her arrange a watering schedule. The student did all the observing and drew her own conclusions. Vocal communication was difficult for this girl and she had little controlled use of her hands. An understanding teacher preserved her autonomy in the experience by simply carrying out according to her desires the parts of the activity she was physically unable to complete. The fact that the activity was carried out as part of an enrichment experience in a *learning center* (SAVI, 1981) with only three students made it much more feasible for the teacher to operate this way. To encourage autonomy on the part of students the teacher should plan in advance, design the instructional experience and facilitate students' autonomy during the learning experience.

The teacher's role during 'input' aspects of the instructional program also focuses on facilitating learning. Carrying out the role, however, includes many activities more traditionally identified as 'teaching'. Input-oriented sessions are effective for a variety of purposes, including introducing new ideas, suggesting a specific laboratory procedure and how to carry it out safely, and helping learners to analyze data and draw conclusions about the evidence they have been collecting. During input sessions a teacher might: (1) introduce new vocabulary; (2) demonstrate how to transfer data to a graph or chart to help highlight trends in the data; (3) introduce a new idea so that students' explorations can be more effective. Careful planning and design of input-oriented sessions is extremely important since teaching is not simply talking, especially if one is working with disabled youngsters and is committed to a multisensory approach to the instructional program. Carefully designed charts and illustrations can help many youngsters understand a point that would totally confuse them if the only input were aural. For those who can see, a well chosen picture can still be worth a thousand words. Giving some youngsters an outline or summary in print or braille can help them to better understand ideas. Using examples from students' recent experiences as the basis for the introduction of new ideas can be extremely helpful. Learning can be considered to take place in cycles and well designed learning cycles usually allow for a period of 'exploration' or familiarity with the general idea or subject before the teacher 'invents' or 'introduces' the new idea during an input session. In the SCIIS program (Thier *et al.*, 1978) can be found a further discussion of the learning cycle and its use in elementary school science. During input sessions the art and showmanship aspects of teaching can come in effectively, as long as the emphasis is on evolving a climate for understanding on the part of the student.

For all students, but especially the disabled, just introducing a new idea cannot be considered adequate to real understanding. Divergent questions (Thier, 1970) that encourage multiple responses can be asked to encourage youngsters to express their own understanding or lack of it. Such questions are successful when they lead to an exchange of ideas and information between youngsters and the teacher or especially between youngsters themselves. Discussions can help individuals to try out and explore their ideas with their peers; here the teacher's role is one of a facilitator rather than immediate provider of right answers. When the input session is designed to pull together data and come to some conclusions the role of the teacher is also very important. He should provide information as effectively as possible, while keeping in mind that teaching can be listening (especially to learners) and learning can be talking, especially as individuals share, reflect on, and revise their ideas in discussions with peers. The *learning center* approach to instruction, with its emphasis on small groups, can contribute significantly to this kind of teaching.

Opportunities for autonomy and input in the experience of learners should be a continuing process. The learner's own (but usually guided) discoveries during autonomous periods lead to and form the basis for new ideas and generalizations introduced by the teaching during input sessions.

These become the organizers for further discovery on the part of learners in sessions that are more autonomous.

Outcomes for Disabled Learners

Our work with the SAVI/SELPH program has shown that experience-based science can contribute to accomplishing significant positive outcomes for disabled learners. Filling-in of experiential gaps, an introduction to scientific and technological devices that can help the individual be more independent, and exposure to career awareness and career opportunities, can all evolve from the disabled learner's study of science. Learning science with its emphasis on evidence-based decision-making can have an impact on disabled individuals and their attitude towards themselves and especially their capabilities.

In science you identify a problem or situation, make observations and collect evidence regarding it. You then use that evidence as the basis for decision-making to solve the problem or change the situation. You then carefully try out your decision and evaluate its effect. Each problem 'solved' or situation 'handled' leads to new understanding and the identification of new problems and situations. This is the nature of science, a continuous exploration of reality using current knowledge and understanding as the basis for questions and investigations leading to increased knowledge and understanding. It is this inquisitive, exploratory, evidence-based attitude that we want to develop in physically disabled individuals. The more the individual can explore and communicate his or her strengths and weak nesses, the more effectively professionals can help the individual cope with the disability. For example, science and technology make it possible for seriously disabled individuals to control a motorized wheel chair using almost any part of their body. Head, foot, hand switches, toggles, pointers, and combinations are in widespread use and provide a degree of independence never thought possible to many individuals. Specific approaches to maximize the individual's capabilities are usually possible if one knows what those capabilities are. If the individual is able to take an evidence-based, investigative approach to determining his or her own capabilities, this can be of enormous help to professionals working with that person. The emphasis here is on a solution, therefore one collects evidence regarding capabilities rather than disabilities. This is the attitude of science which can instil in the disabled individual an attitude of focusing on what one can do and how that can be applied, thus helping the individual cope with the disability. Not all problems are as amenable to solution as that of controlling a wheelchair. The more we can instil in disabled individuals this inquisitive, investigative, experience and evidence-based attitude that is science, the more they can cope with their disabilities and find ways to emphasize their capabilities.

Science experiences can also have a significant impact on the interaction of young disabled individuals with their non-disabled peers (MacDougall *et al.*, 1980). Hands-on activity provides a new experience that the disabled and non-disabled learner can share. Adaptations need to be made so that disabled learners can participate along with their non-disabled peers. Our research in the classroom (Chiba and Thier, 1982) shows that such experiences increase positive interactions between disabled and non-disabled learners and build a cooperative atmosphere in the mainstreamed classroom.

Science experiences can have positive effects on the attitudes of disabled individuals to themselves and their interaction with non-disabled peers. Such experiences can also contribute significantly to related learning by disabled individuals. The emphasis on making observations and collecting evidence can easily lead to increased use of oral and written language as one describes one's observations and evidence to peers and others. When conclusions are drawn, their basis and justification need to be communicated to others in oral or written form. This provides an opportunity for language development and enrichment. The fact that the focus is on what took place during the collection of evidence makes it easier for disabled individuals to participate in the discussion. Since so much of science is based on the collection, comparison, and analysis of quantitative data, many opportunities for the use of mathematics become available and these can be used to teach new skills.

In a hands-on experience-based science program opportunities abound for learning and reinforcing skills in everyday life, ranging from the use of a screw-driver to how to measure and pour liquids and powders. The emphasis can be on maximizing the individual's capabilities rather than highlighting their disabilities. These and a wide variety of other possibilities for providing meaningful learning experiences in the broadest definition of the term become possible when a hands-on materials-centered science program is an integral part of the overall educational experience of disabled learners. Such programs can also help the disabled individual learn how to collect and analyze the data necessary to monitor their own adaptations to various conditions. This can be extremely helpful in fostering better health through adaptive behaviour.

References

BREDDERMAN, T. (1982) 'What research says', *Science and Children*, National Science Teachers Association, Washington, D.C., September.

CHIBA, C. and THIER, H.D. (1982) *The Impact of a Multisensory Science Program on the Social Interactions of Disabled Children*. C.M.L. Lawrence Hall of Science, University of California, Berkeley, Calif.

HARMS, N. and YAGER, R.E. (1981) 'What research says to the science teacher', *National Science Teachers Association Monograph*, Vol. 3, Washington, D.C.

HAWKINS, D., (1969) 'Messing about in science', *Science and Children*, II, February,

Herbert D. Thier (USA)

pp. 5–9.

HEALTH ACTIVITIES PROJECT (HAP) (1980) Lawrence Hall of Science, Northbrook, Ill., Hubbard Publishers.

KARPLUS, R., (1981) 'Response by the Oersted Medalist: Autonomy and input', *American Journal of Physics*, 49, 9, pp. 811–14.

MACDOUGALL, A. *et al.* (1980) 'The use of activity-centered science activities to facilitate mainstreaming', Deans Project, School of Education, University of Michigan, Ann Arbor, Mich.

SAVI (1981) *Leadership Trainers Manual*, C.M.L. Lawrence Hall of Science, University of California, Berkeley, Calif.

SAVI/SELPH (1981) Further information about the SAVI/SELPH program is available from C.M.L., Lawrence Hall of Science, University of California, Berkeley, Calif.

STAKE, R. E. and EASLEY, J., JR (1978) *Case Studies in Science Education*, Washington, D.C., US Government Printing Office.

THIER, H.D. (1970) *Teaching Elementary Science: A Laboratory Approach*, D.C. Heath and Company, pp. 123–61.

THIER, H.D. *et al.* (1978) 'Subsystems and variables', or other units of the Rand McNally Revision of the SCIC Programs XVIII-XIX, currently published by Delta Education.

TYLER, G. (1982) 'The American High School Today and Tomorrow', address at a conference, University of California, Berkeley, Calif.

VOSS, B.E. (1983) 'Student achievements: Curriculum teaching strategy effects', University of Michigan.

A Programme of Nutritional Education in Outlying Areas of Spain with a High Incidence of Goitre

Pilar Najera

Nutritional problems in Spain are few; general knowledge on nutrition is good, due mostly to the Food and Nutrition Education Programme (Education en Alimentacion y Nutricion — Programa EDALNU) which started in 1962, with assistance from UNICEF, WHO and FAO. Nevertheless, in some underdeveloped, mountainous areas of the country endemic goitre is a problem, affecting 13.4 per cent of adults and from 56 to 80 per cent of schoolchildren. The main aetiological factors are the lack or scarcity of iodine and the ingestion of goitrogens which contaminate water and food. Action to mitigate this situation has emphasized changes in eating habits through health education (balanced diet, use of salt supplemented with iodine and selected foods) and agricultural extension to modify local agricultural traditions through the introduction of new vegetables.

Identification, Description and Analysis

The existence of endemic goitre and cretinism has been known since 1927, and several limited initiatives had been taken in some areas (Hurdes, Alpujarras) achieving some reduction in goitre rates. However, no comprehensive plan had been envisaged until the present one. This entailed summarizing all available information on the subject, with special studies on presence of iodine in drinking water and soil; incidence of iodine in urine and blood; direct and indirect consumption of salt (amount and type); medical examination of schoolchildren (re their physical and mental development); surveys on food consumption.

The data indicated an environmental deficiency in iodine in wide areas of the country, particularly in some mountainous areas. Communication difficulties have kept these populations isolated and self-contained. In these 'high risk' areas, it has also been found that: (1) the concentration of iodine in urine is so low as to increase the probability of the presence of cases of cretinism (urinary excretion of iodine of 15–30 ug/day in schoolchildren of Atienza-Guadalajara); (2) the height and weight of schoolchildren are below the regional mean figures; (3) there is a delay in bone development; and (4) there are deficiencies in intellectual and psychomotor development.

A psychometric study has been done in several of these areas, evaluating intellectual and psychomotor level, degree of perception, motor rapidity and visual memory. The results were below the normal mean in tests with standardized values for the Spanish population. Some tests have been specially prepared for this population, and at the moment the study of a comparative control group of areas with similar problems (isolation, rural agricultural life, etc.) but no goitre is taking place, in order to eliminate the bias due to the socio-cultural environment.

The study of food consumption verified what was already known from former studies: enormous monotony of the diet; daily ingestion of vegetables of the genus *Brassica* (cabbage cauliflower, turnip, etc.); and very little consumption of fish, molluscs and other foods rich in iodine. These areas are: the mountainous districts of Las Hurdes, Sierra de Guadalajara, Alpujarras (Sierra Nevada), Ancares and smaller mountainous areas in Santander, Sierra de Segura and others.

To control this situation a national plan of action was formulated, including a programme of health education in nutrition, which would make a particularly important contribution. The objectives of this educational programme were as follows:

1 *For the whole country:*
   reinforcement and wider diffusion of knowledge about a balanced diet and ways of getting it by means of an adequate range and combination of foods;
   information on iodine deficiency in many areas of the country and of the advantage of using iodine salt instead of common salt. The idea of substitution has been stressed, making it clear that it is important not to increase the amount of salt in foods.
2 *For 'high risk' areas:*
   to ensure in school and adult populations a basic knowledge of food and nutrition;
   to stimulate the consumption of specific foods not traditionally used, especially (or at least) by children and the use of salt supplemented with iodine;
   to make the population understand the influence of an unvarying diet and of the intensive use of goitrogen foods, and the association with goitre and the delay in the development and achievement of children;
   to inculcate in teachers, health professionals and other technical personnel in the community a level of knowledge consistent with their previous training, their functions and their educational poten-

tial about endemic goitre and its causes, and ways of preventing it; to stimulate participation in this plan of every person in the community who, through status or personal circumstances, can contribute. These people must know the objectives of the plan and their the role, and must be ready to collaborate in its implementation and evaluation.

Policies, Strategies and Methods

The plan implies coordination of a series of actions, among which an important place is occupied by the health education programme. These actions are: elaboration of a technical norm for the addition of iodine to salt; production and marketing of iodine salt; development of the commercial infrastructure needed to introduce this product to the goitrous areas which are difficult of access due to physical and social isolation; introduction of new foods to these areas; and participation of autonomous regions, i.e., the self-governing regions that now constitute the Spanish state; continuation of studies of naturally-occurring goitrogens and their presence in water, soil and sedimentary rocks. The plan has already been developed in several phases.

Preparatory Phase

During this phase studies were developed to find out that type of salt (by degree of humidity and size of grain) which must be supplemented with iodine. This is important because in these areas many types of sausages and salted meats are prepared at home using types of salt other than table salt. Other studies were carried out to determine the chemical to employ in supplementation, its dosage and standardized procedures for analysis and control.

The first educational activity was to interest manufacturers and managers of salt packing and distribution enterprises in the preparation of iodine supplemented salt, and to enlist their cooperation in order to improve distribution networks in mountainous and inaccessible areas. During this first phase audiovisual materials were prepared which would be used in conjunction with the programme.

Health authorities of the autonomous regions were co-opted into the overall plan and charged with acting in 'high risk' areas. Health personnel in goitre-prone areas were involved in the programme; the need for integrated community action was stressed. It is important to underline the sensitization of health and education personel during earlier field studies, since they were present during the activities of medical and psychological terms and in many cases cooperated in the development of the studies.

Pilar Najera (Spain)

Action Phase

This phase comprises several stages.

Stage 1. *Informing key personnel*

Information for teachers and other personnel in 'high risk' areas on goitre, its causes and prevention and incentives for their active participation in the programme of health education for schoolchildren. To assist them a publication, 'Technical information for teachers', will be distributed. This booklet covers content and methods for understanding the subject and includes suggestions on teaching materials.

Information for health personnel (family doctors, school doctors,* pharmacists, veterinarians, nurses and midwives) in the areas where the programme is to be developed intensively through distribution of the WHO publication, 'Fight against endemic goitre'. Their cooperation will be enlisted in the training of teachers, and they will have a very special role as resource personnel.

Information for agricultural extension service agents on the objectives and content of the plan and the programmes that will be introduced or improved in each area. They will use the same material as the teachers because they have many educational tasks among the population. Nearly all these agents have had elementary training in nutritional education through the EDALNU courses and nearly a third of them have advanced training to diploma level.

Every person who is going to participate in these educational activities will be equipped with a series of slides on the subject, two different posters on balanced diet and 'supplemented salt' and leaflets for additional information for the people.

Stage 2. *An information campaign through the mass media:*

Televising two publicity films to promote goitre prevention through a balanced diet and the use of salt supplemented with iodine.

Broadcasting radio messages nationally and locally, with local broadcasting concentrating on the 'high risk' areas.

In addition to the organized programme, local health authorities have been asked to use other media (newspapers, etc.), bearing in mind the characteristics of the target population and the best ways of reaching it.

Stage 3. *Intensification of dissemination of information in the community*, employing appropriate reinforcement techniques for rural populations, to comment on and explain the information received through television, radio, newspapers, etc. The involvement of grocers and mobile shops (in outlying parts)

*In Spain the number of school doctors is very small. By law in small places the duties of school doctors must be undertaken by family doctors.

through the distribution of stickers, leaflets and distinctive signs where iodine supplemented salt and other recommended foods can be found is considered particularly important. The sale of fried and fresh fish, dairy products, etc. is also being promoted. The use of dried cod is widespread in Spain in rural and urban areas and there are many traditional ways of cooking it. This is a practice easy to introduce in 'high risk' areas.

Special reference must be made to the teaching activities of the agricultural extension services. *Male agents* are specially trained to teach farmers about improvements in agriculture, use of fertilizers and pesticides; their work is directed to the established farmer, and, as a special task, the training of young men in agriculture. *Female agents* work with housewives in the improvement of home life, including the diet and use of farm and natural products. In this programme their main task is teaching about a balanced diet in which meals are prepared with products from the local area or with foreign products easily and cheaply obtainable, and suggesting menus and recipes where fresh or preserved fish are included.

This programme of health education has the following features:

cooperation of industrial and commercial salt sectors with the health administration;

participation of the agricultural extension service, which has maintained a close relationship with the public health services from the beginning of the EDALNU programme. Its collaboration has been necessary and highly effective in rural areas where other community development agents are lacking;

coordination of the mass media campaigns with educational activities, especially at the level of person to person, and of teachers and health personnel in the community. This is especially true of the 'high risk' areas;

overall, unified action by teachers and health personnel, local and provincial, which was developed during earlier studies; this exemplifies the idea of community action developed through open discussion and popular participation.

Progress Report and Evaluation

The plan has now reached the end of the preparatory phase: all the specifications for iodine supplemented salt are ready and in the hands of the industries that are preparing the product; all the audiovisual media are ready; personnel of the agricultural extension services at national level have been involved in the programme, as have authorities of the autonomous regions. An evaluation has been planned and can be summarized as follows:

1 Evaluation of administrative action
Every item of the scheduled activities of this preliminary phase has been accomplished as per plan with very few exceptions. The materials are ready for distribution and the personnel committed. Less successful has been the participation of certain autonomous regions due mostly to the lesser degree to which their populations are affected. Health authorities of the Basque Government are not participating because in their territory the amount of goitre is not enough to be considered a high priority in relation to other health responsibilities. Economic support for the programme has been obtained through special funds for the prevention of subnormality.

2 Evaluation of the information and education programmes
This will be done by reference to the:
number of leaflets, posters, and stickers used by teachers, health and agricultural personnel;
number of lessons, talks, conferences, group discussions and any other information initiatives developed and the audience (number and type);
number of people reached by TV and radio at different times of broadcast messages;
surveys, through a simple questionnaire, to find out the impact of the mass media (number of questionnaires completed and study of the answers);
number of specific requests made to the population.

3 In the medium term (a year after the beginning of the action phase): a study of the nutritional knowledge of schoolchildren; a survey of new varieties of vegetables introduced into the area and new species of farm animals; a survey of new food products in the market; an estimate of the increase in the sale of iodine supplemented salt.

4 In the long term (after five years): a survey of the increase in the mean weight and height of children; a survey of the improved performance of children of the same age using the original tests; a study of thyroid glands of schoolchildren at the start (6 years old) and finish (14 years old) of school (number of children and degree of goitre); indications of other signs of personal and social development in the area (increase in the number of adolescents entering secondary or professional education, number of industries, shops, etc. opened).

Reduction in the incidence and prevalence of goitre is very important. However, this plan is also intended to promote the social and cultural development of these areas. Iodine supplementation is important, but more is expected of the elimination or reduction of the use of some goitrogen vegetables and of the introduction of a wider variety of foods for a balanced diet.

Health Education and Initial Teacher Training in England and Wales

Trefor Williams

Whenever health education is discussed in relationship to schools the question of initial teacher education is raised. Most of the reports of international organizations concerned directly or indirectly with health education (UNESCO, WHO) make recommendations concerning the inclusion of health education as an important element of the pre-service education of teachers.

In England and Wales there has been, in colleges of education at least, a tradition of health education which stretches back to the beginning of the century. Such a tradition has not been so marked in the Postgraduate Certificate in Education Courses. The traditions of health education courses seem to have diminished markedly since the early to mid-60s with the advent of BEd courses and the accent on academic courses of study. Health education appeared to have declined in the late 1970s to the point where it no longer commanded any standing in teacher education. The paradox of this situation was that while on the decline in teacher education courses, there appeared to be a distinct upsurge of health education activity in schools which now recognized its importance and relevance to children and young people. Early in 1981 the Health Education Council invited the Health Education Unit, University of Southampton, to undertake a research and development project to discover what was really happening regarding health education in initial teacher education and to develop strategies and materials for its re-establishment as a viable and important part of the professional preparation of teachers.

The study included three major investigations:

1 a national survey of schools in England and Wales;
2 a national survey of initial teacher education courses in England and Wales;
3 a national study of initial teacher students in England and Wales.

This paper will concentrate mainly upon the survey of initial teacher education institutions, although it will make reference first to the national survey of schools which provides a context for the whole study.

A National Survey of School Health Education

The survey consisted of a postal questionnaire sent to a $12\frac{1}{2}$ per cent random sample of all primary and secondary state schools in England and Wales. The purpose was:

1   to determine what and how health education is being taught in primary and secondary schools;
2   what part headteachers and senior teachers think health education should play in the initial training of teachers.

The report of this survey (unpublished) was presented to the Health Education Council in spring 1982. The results of the survey (see Table 1) showed that health education was included in the curriculum of the great majority of schools and that headteachers and senior teachers believed strongly that health education should be included in the pre-service education of teachers.

Table 1.   *Health Education in Schools: Selected Data from the Schools Survey*

(Overall response rate to the questionnaire was 76 per cent)

91 per cent of all schools teach or have plans to teach health education
31 per cent of primary schools have a planned programme
69 per cent of secondary schools have a planned programme
18 per cent of primary schools have a designated person for health education
49 per cent of secondary schools have a designated person for health education
98 per cent of primary schools use outside agencies in their health education programme
97 per cent of secondary schools use outside agencies in their health education programme
47 per cent of primary schools use televised health education programmes
43 per cent of secondary schools use televised health education programmes
93 per cent of all schools either strongly agree or agree that schools have a responsibility to teach health education
98 per cent of respondents strongly agree or agree that initial teacher education should include a core programme of health education for all students

The questionnaire also contained questions related to the context and organization of health education in both schools and pre-service courses for teachers.

The evidence available suggests that health education is being taught in the schools of England and Wales although the real extent and quality is impossible to gauge from this survey. It is evidence enough, however, to suggest that student teachers should at the very least be sensitized to the health education needs of pupils and its relationship to their own teaching and the school curriculum.

Health Education in Initial Teacher Education

The second phase of the study was directed at pre-service teaching courses. There are two possible avenues to teacher status in England and Wales:

1 a three or four-year course leading to the professional qualification of Bachelor of Education (BEd). These courses are usually to be found in colleges of higher education.

2 a one-year postgraduate course leading to the Postgraduate Certificate in Education (PGCE). These courses are usually found in the departments or schools of education in universities or polytechnics.

After a false start involving the piloting of a large and unwieldy questionnaire, it was decided to tackle the investigation in three phases:

1 a simple one-page questionnaire to establish basic facts on whether or not health education was included in the teacher education course and, if so, its context, and secondly, to establish contact with a colleague in each of the institutions;

2 visits to about one-third of the institutions and interviews with the named contact;

3 a postal inquiry to all institutions based upon information discovered in phases 1 and 2 concerning the best avenues for health education and the range and kind of materials which might be required.

The First Tentative Inquiry

The first one-page questionnaire was sent out in March 1982 to the Head of the Education Department in each of the teacher education institutions. The response was good and from the returns it was possible to make a very tentative assessment of where health education stood in relation to teacher education generally in England, Wales and Northern Ireland (see tables 2 and 3).

From this data it will be seen that only 24 per cent of institutions

Table 2.   Health Education in Initial Teacher Education: Responses to First Questionnaire

Type of establishment	Number sent	Number returned	As percentage
Colleges of Higher Education	55	50	91
Departments of Education — Polytechnics	26	23	88
Departments of Education — Universities	23	20	87
Total	104	93	89

Table 3. Number of Institutions Where Health Education Is Included

Type of establishment	Health education included		As core for all		As option for some		Both option and core	
	No.	%	No.	%	No.	%	No.	%
Colleges of Higher Education	37	74	12	24	22	44	3	6
Departments of Education — Polytechnics	14	61	8	35	4	17	2	9
Departments of Education — Universities	8	40	2	10	5	25	1	5
Total	59	63	22	24	31	33	6	6

include health education as a *requirement* for all students, but as many as 63 per cent of institutions include a health education component somewhere in their courses either as an option or a core. It begs the questions of the quantity (time given to health education) and the quality of the work being carried out but, nevertheless, it does offer some measure of the interest to be found in the institutions. What is disappointing — and perhaps it was a disappointment to be expected in the light of the time available for the total programme — is the relatively low number of university departments which offer a small core of health education for their students. Even this low figure of 10 per cent needs to be treated with some caution as it gives a false sense of the importance accorded to health education which in some PGCE courses will consist of a one-hour general lecture in health education. What is encouraging is that a third of all institutions offer an option course in health education. Although such courses vary considerably in terms of time allowance, scope and content, they show a desire on the part of institutions and teaching staff to provide opportunities for students to consider the implications of health education for their own teaching.

Context of the Health Education Input

It is difficult to clårify the context in which health education is presented from this first tentative questionnaire, but because the context in which it is to be used is important for an understanding of the kind and background of materials to be developed it is useful to attempt to do so here. There are, however, at least three important background points to be borne in mind while considering the data:

1 the lack of common structures to initial teacher education courses which is particularly emphasized in contrasting PGCE and BEd courses;

2 lack of a precise and common terminology in describing context, e.g., Educational Studies, Professional Studies, Curricular Studies;

3   in some instances health education will occur under several contextual headings in the same institution, e.g., Educational Studies, Primary School Science and Curricular Studies.

For these reasons the responses have been quantified so as to provide a rank order of the contexts within which health education appears (see Tables 4 and 5). The ranking is based upon the number of times a particular 'context' is mentioned as providing a medium for health education. (This number will not correspond to the number of institutions because many mentioned several different contexts within which health education will occur.)

Table 4.   Context for Health Education (Number of Times Mentioned)

	Colleges	Polytechnics	Universities	Total	Rank order
Professional Studies	14	2	2	18	1
Science	5	4	4	13	2
Separate Core/Option	9	3	1	13	2
Educational Studies	6	4	1	11	4
First Aid	4	0	2	6	5
Curriculum Studies	3	1	1	5	6
Special Education	4	0	0	4	7
Physical Education	1	2	0	3	8
Health and Safety	2	1	0	3	8

Table 5.   Ranking of Contexts by Type of Institution

Colleges	1. Professional Studies 2. Separate Course 3. Education Studies 4. Science
Polytechnics	1. Science: Education Studies 3. Separate Course 4. Professional Studies: PE
Universities	1. Science 2. First Aid 3. Separate Course: Educational Studies: Curriculum Studies

While it would be rash to draw a definitive conclusion from these rankings, it is worth noting them as a useful background against which whatever materials are needed can be developed. As well as providing a useful guide to the planning of materials which will have exposure to all students, it is a good indicator of the specialist subject interest, e.g., sciences (particularly biology) and physical education. It is also a reminder of the need to help those college courses which do provide a *separate* course in health education for their students.

Phase 2 and 3 of the Study

These phases of the study were closely interlinked and for this reason are reported together. Phase 2 consisted of an interview of approximately one-third of colleagues identified from the first questionnaire, while Phase 3 consisted of a postal questionnaire to all institutions which sought to verify and further clarify the findings of Phase 2. The interviews were conducted in thirty-three of the 104 institutions concerned with initial teacher education as follows:

Colleges of Education	15
Polytechnic Departments of Education	7
University Departments of Education	11
Total	33

The questionnaires were sent to all teacher education institution (104) and the response rate was 82 per cent (eighty-five institutions). Space does not allow a detailed report on each of these phases of the project so I have selected some of the main issues and data from both.

Best Avenues for Health Education

Interviews. The interviews of tutors had emphasized the difficulty of placing or enlarging a health education input into an already overcrowded curriculum for pre-service teacher training. Because of this much of the interview time was spent considering the most useful ways (avenues) in which health education could be introduced or developed. The views of tutors can be summarized as falling into several categories:

(1) *Separate course* — a minority of tutors, particulary in the colleges, were keen to retain or develop a separate course in health education. In the context of the majority of institutions, however, this would present difficulties because of (i) shortage of available curriculum time; (ii) lack of experienced and qualified staff; (iii) need to include plan for validating bodies.

(2) *In education course* — this possibility was quite popular with the colleges. It was argued that if students see it as part of education they will recognize it as being important. One tutor remarked that health education ought to permeate the whole curriculum but *must* be significant in educational courses because it presented relevant issues for students to consider, research, discuss and attempt to solve.

(3) *Through professional course and 'main subject' studies* — those concerned with PGCE courses tended to favour the introduction of health education through a professional course related to the preparation for teaching — usually of a specific subject area. Most of the health education being

attempted in university departments, for example, is currently through professional studies related to the preparation of science (biology) teachers. In the colleges also it was suggested that health education could well be developed in the context of some main subject studies. Areas with considerable potential for development here were suggested: science — biology; home economics; primary school science; physical education.

(4) *Options* — there was general agreement that both PGCE and BEd courses might include an optional course for students in health education. Important considerations here would be: (i) work at the student's own level; (ii) work related to teaching in schools; (iii) introduction to students of pupil materials and appropriate methodologies.

(5) *A health education core for all* — all tutors felt that a core for all students was a desirable aim but there was some difficulty in seeing how it might be possible. Possibilities suggested were: within an education course, perhaps particularly associated with child growth and development; as a separate and discrete health education course either as a 'course' over several weeks or in terms or as an 'immersion' course providing an intensive exposure to health education during one or two days.

Questionnaire. The questions relating to possible avenues for health education sought mainly to confirm and clarify the possibilities available to institutions as follows:

1   In response to the question: Do you agree that it would be useful to produce materials appropriate to Education and/or Professional Studies? the respondents replied as follows:

Type of institution	Educational Studies		Professional Studies	
	Yes	No	Yes	No
Colleges	32	—	38	—
Polytechnics	11	—	10	—
Universities	17	—	20	—
Total	60	—	68	—

71 per cent of respondents felt it appropriate to develop health education materials within the context of Educational Studies (n = 85); 80 per cent of respondents felt it appropriate to develop health education materials within the context of Professional Studies (n = 85).

2   82 per cent of respondents agreed that it would be useful to develop materials which help relate health education to several subject areas.

In indicating which would be the three most appropriate subject areas suitable for links with health education, the following views were expressed:

Institution	Biology	PE	Home Economics	RE	General Science	Other
Colleges	31	26	24	20	17	4
Polytechnics	7	7	7	3	6	1
Universities	12	12	13	9	13	1
Total	54	45	44	32	36	6

Biology (54), physical education (45) and home economics (44) were the three specialist subject areas most frequently mentioned as being the most appropriate to be associated with health education.

Materials for the Promotion of Health Education in Teacher Education. The interviews had shown up a severe lack of materials specifically written for use in pre-service courses for teachers. Tutors tended to use a variety of sources for student readings and discussions and were warmly in favour of (1) a short text written specifically for student teachers; and (2) workshop materials in specific areas.

Student Text. It was clear from discussions with tutors that there were no texts or books which were written specifically for students. Most mentioned the materials available from school health education projects as a prime source (5–13, 13–18, TACADE, Lifeskills, Active Tutorial, etc.). Generally it was felt that a student-oriented text would be a useful and practical addition to the available materials. This view was supported by responses to the questionnaire: 93 per cent (seventy-nine institutions) of respondents would find a student text useful; 89 per cent (seventy-six institutions) of respondents would certainly use it.

Workshop Materials. There was also general agreement amongst those interviewed on the need for materials which would promote discussion, investigation, reflection and in other ways involve the students with health education. One tutor summed up the feeling of most colleagues when he said: 'The materials need to be challenging, participatory and thought provoking.' A challenge indeed! The materials would also need to embody the kind of teaching and learning strategies which were suggested for use in schools, and in this sense might provide 'models' for the students' own practice with their pupils. A third point mentioned repeatedly was the need to link whatever 'thought provoking' materials for students that might be developed with materials currently available for pupils in schols. Many tutors emphasized the need for student-oriented materials to remain as flexible as possible so that they might be used in the context of the many possible avenues already outlined.

The need for such materials was also reflected in replies to the questionnaires: 84 per cent (seventy-one institutions) of respondents reported that discussion promoting materials in health education would be likely to be used in their institutions in one or other of the contexts referred to earlier. Respondents were asked to list specific topic areas which would be most useful in the context of workshop materials; the following represents a ranking of topics according to the number of times they were mentioned:

1 Drugs
2 Diet, Sex Education, Safety
5 Smoking, Relationships
7 Alcohol
8 Sexuality
9 Self-Image, Pollution.

A Summary and Plan for Action

General

The first observation refers to the difficulty of getting 'health education' into the curricula of initial teacher education courses. The best strategies seem to be to infiltrate courses through as many different avenues as possible. This means, however, that the materials produced will need to be flexible. Education or professional studies courses seem to be the best avenues to follow if health education is to reach *all* students.

Specific

The evidence from the investigation to date suggests the following courses of action:

1 the development of an attractive 'base line' text for students;
2 the development of health education 'workshop' materials which would be aimed at the student's own level but which would also connect with available school-based material;
3 the development of health education materials specifically related to specialist subject areas, e.g., biology, home economics, physical education, primary school science;
4 the development of a tutor's guide to facilitate the planning of 'health education' inputs or courses as appropriate to the needs of students and the time available;
5 to provide some means by which tutors can become familiar with the materials so as to facilitate their use in pre-service courses.

Trial Interprofessional Workshop Courses in School and Community Health Education

George Campbell

The workshop has arrived, if by 'workshop' is meant an individually or group-centred learning experience which is perhaps the very antithesis of the experience of the passive recipient of a mass lecture. The workshop has clearly defined but limited objectives (limited in the sense of being attainable either immediately or in the short term). Furthermore, the associated learning process is seen to be relevant to a working situation, it builds on the experience of the participant and usually has immediate practical outcomes as well as long-term benefits. The workshop also actively involves the participants in a carefully graduated series of tasks. In-service courses which involve workshop sessions are increasingly seen by participants to be of value to them, and such courses where they are imaginatively planned and carefully organized are deservedly well supported.

Between November 1981 and March 1982 the Family Planning Association organized a series of three workshop courses in Basingstoke, Hampshire. The purpose was to bring together the members of different professions and agencies involved in one particularly sensitive area of the secondary school health education curriculum: sexuality and personal relationships education. It was hoped that the participants would acquire knowledge and skills which would enhance the quality of their work in this area with young people. In addition, the opportunities presented by a carefully planned series of workshop sessions over three days might promote a desire to continue to work together after the course in spite of such practical difficulties as heavy workloads, tight timetables and contrasting work patterns and styles.

The significance of these particular courses in interprofessional work lay only partly in their aims and methodology, since similar initiatives have been occurring in various parts of Britain. Of considerable importance was the unusual feature that they were to be closely monitored at every possible point and evaluated — a process extending from the planning stage to the post-course period

The evaluation[1] was conducted as rigorously as circumstances permitted. What was achieved was a detailed daily profile of each three-day course, with a retrospective view taken within ten days of the end of each course and again several months later.

The Basingstoke Initiative: Background and Rationale

Basingstoke, while not possessing the chronic problems of inner-city areas of large conurbations has, nevertheless, certain difficulties. It is an older 'new town' with a relatively recent history of large-scale immigration from London, a large school population which is contributing to an already high proportion of unemployed and an accentuation of 'home problems', and, in consequence, the greater involvement of various professional caring services.

For several years the Family Planning Association (FPA) Centre in Basingstoke has provided short in-service courses for those involved in sex education in the community and in schools. The experimental series proposed by the local FPA Education Officer were to be multidisciplinary, three in number, each identical in content and organization and each centred on a group of secondary schools and their catchments. It was hoped to recruit teachers, education welfare officers, health visitors, doctors, school nurses, social workers and youth and community workers who were located in the same school catchment or district.

The purpose of each course was to give an introduction to the subject of sex education, and over a three day-period to provide basic information and 'opportunities to consider various aspects of human sexuality and relationships including experience of different methods of exploring and communicating ideas and feelings on these subjects.' Through a workshop approach using experiential methods of learning, the members of different professional groups could thus together bring to bear their particular disciplinary perspectives in a series of group tasks designed to increase understanding of sexuality and personal relationships education.

The FPA invited the University of Southampton Department of Education, which had been involved in a previous interagency research and development project in Hampshire, to evaluate the series. The cooperation of local officers of the health, medical, social and educational services and elected members was enlisted; then the local schools were formally invited to participate. A meeting addressed by the FPA organizers on the subject of the course and by the university representatives on the evaluation was well attended by officials, teachers and members of community agencies. Elected members were unable to attend. The timing of the meeting was important in that it followed the local SCHEP Stage 2 Workshop which was well supported by teachers (and attended by an evaluator), and local interest generally in school health educational developments seemed to be increasing. Support at the meeting for the experimental courses was evident and plans were set in motion for an autumn 1981 start.

Course Aims and Objectives

The aims and objectives were as stated in the FPA's programme for each of the three courses:

Overall aim:
> To help course members to be more sensitive, confident and comfortable in working with young people in the area of sexuality and personal relationships.

During and as a result of this course, participants should expect:—
  (i) to acquire some facts about sexuality and to be aware of relevant sources for more information;
 (ii) to identify feelings, attitudes and values about sexuality of self and others;
(iii) to appreciate the feelings, attitudes and values that others might have towards sexuality;
 (iv) to be more aware of the needs of young people with regard to sex education;
  (v) to gain insight into the areas of sexuality and sex education covered by other professions/agencies and to be more aware of their approaches, values and methods;
 (vi) to feel willing to cooperate and give mutual support to these other professions and agencies

After the course members might expect to show an increased ability in the following skills:
  (i) communicating about sexuality and personal relationships;
 (ii) developing discussion with pupils/clients/young people on their attitudes and feelings about sexuality and personal relationships.

Course Participants: Numbers and Occupations

In spite of determined efforts on the part of the organizers to recruit two from each of the main occupational groups, this balance was not fully achieved. Certain important groups were unrepresented: general practitioners, police and the district health education officer (who was on secondment). Of the thirty-six participants, thirty volunteered to attend, six did not (the latter were doctors (three), health visitors (two), intermediate treatment officer (one). The pattern of recruitment to the three courses is set out in Table 1.

Table 1.   Recruitment to the Courses

	Course 1	Course 2	Course 3	Total
Teachers	5	3	3	11
Education welfare officers (EWOs)	2	2	1	5
Health visitors	1	1	2	4
Doctors school doctors / clinical medical officers	2	—	2	4
School nurses	—	2	2	4
Social workers	2	—	1	3
Further education lecturers	—	—	2	2
School matron	—	—	1	1
Intermediate treatment officer	—	—	1	1
Community service volunteer	—	1	—	1
Total	12	9	15	36

Course Participants: Experience

1   *Work with the age group 11–18:* thirty out of thirty-six. Excluded were four health visitors and two social workers. The average number of years worked with the age group was six.

2   *Contact with schools and/or colleges:* thirty-six out of thirty-six, thirty-one being connected with a particular institution or group of institutions.

3   *Contact with other professions or agencies.* Most participants recorded some contact with at least one other professional group. The most frequently identified were: first, social worker and general practitioner; second, teacher, education welfare officer and careers officers; third, probation officer, school doctor and police; fourth, health visitor, educational psychologist, hospital consultant and school nurse. Six out of the ten professions or agencies represented on the courses were mentioned. Conversely, relatively highly placed in the first and second groups of contacts were professions or agencies not represented on the courses: general practitioner and careers officer.

4   *Involvement in sex education.* Participants differed greatly in the extent to which they thought they were already involved in the sex education of young people. Nine of the eleven teachers felt that they had quite a strong involvement, not only in programmed courses but also in personal counselling, which may occur within or outside the tutorial system. This also applied to the two further education lecturers. Two teachers felt that their involvement was limited,

consisting only of teaching a small part of a wider course. Of the five
EWOs, two gave no reply to this question, two considered their
involvement minimal or non-existent, and one saw it as giving
advice to individual children as the need arose. The four health
visitors in the main saw their involvement as minimal; two considered it non-existent. One had been involved in three sessions on
sex education in schools in the last six months, but her main work
was with unmarried mothers and girls who have terminations.
Another ran a course, one night a week, on preparation for
parenthood which had a component of sex and personal relationships education. The four school nurses also thought their
involvement minimal or nil. One expressed dissatisfaction with this
situation, stating that she would like to be involved more. The four
doctors' opinions of their involvement differed: two considered
their involvement virtually nil, while the other two saw it in terms of
counselling and giving information. The three social workers, the
intermediate treatment officer and community service volunteer saw
their involvement mainly as counselling individual clients. The
school matron saw her involvement as one-to-one counselling,
timetabled or spontaneous discussion with small groups of children,
consultation in development of school programme for health/sex
education for first to third years. She was also invited into the
classroom for general discussin or to view and discuss various films.
Participants were also asked whether they had any previous experience of FPA courses. Eleven had attended such courses, but only
four of them on education courses in the last two or three years. The
majority (seven out of eleven) were members of course 3.

Participants' Expectations of the Course

Intending participants were given a list of course objectives and asked in
which three areas they hoped to be helped most:

1 knowledge about sexuality;
2 clarification of one's own feelings, attitudes, values about sexuality;
3 appreciation of the feelings, attitudes, values of others about
   sexuality;
4 awareness of the needs of young people with regard to sex education;
5 insight into the areas of sexuality covered by other professions/
   agencies;
6 cooperation between professions/agencies;
7 ability in communicating about sexuality;
8 ability in developing discussion about sexuality.

There were thirty-five replies. The strongest preferences were for those objectives concerned with greater awareness of young people's feelings and the development of communication skills. Less than half showed a preference for 'appreciating others' feelings towards sexuality' or 'gaining insight into the work of other professions/agencies'. The smallest proportion (one in nine) showed a preference for developing cooperation between professions/agencies.

Participants' Views of the Composition of the Group on Each of the Three Courses

On all courses while participants welcomed the range of professions/agencies present, they were critical of the absence of others whom they considered ought to have attended, especially those attached to a particular school. A wider range would have been preferred, particularly on courses 1 and 2 where only five different occupational groups were represented compared with nine on course 3. On all courses the additional professions/agencies specifically requested were:

social workers	6 requests
	(all from course 2 which had none)
probation officers	3 requests
marriage/family guidance	3 requests
police	2 requests
general practitioners	2 requests

The small number of men on the courses was a criticism of twenty-five of the thirty-six participants. There was one man on each of Courses 1 and 2, and two on Course 3. Members felt that the male input was limited, that there were not enough men to provide a balance, and that discussions lacked a male viewpoint. However, as two participants commented, 'It might have been useful in discussion if there had been more men, but the composition was probably representative of those concerned with the sex education of young people, i.e. more women then men.'

On Course 2 two participants thought that the age range did not seem wide enough; the group was lacking in the younger viewpoint as most of the group were married women with children.

The Three Courses: Content and Approach

Over each of the three-day periods there were fourteen workshop sessions devoted to opening up new ground in sex and personal relationships education. There were, in addition, review sessions which occurred at the beginning and end of each day. Each of the fourteen sessions was well defined with clearly stated objectives and methods set out in tutors' notes. At the commencement of most sessions the objectives and method of working were explained. At the end of each session there was usually a plenary discussion devoted to reviewing and sharing what had been experienced and learnt.

At the end the course there was a session devoted to reviewing the overall experience. Participants were invited to consider whether the course had helped them to (1) appreciate young people's needs and feelings in sex education, and (2) feel more able to meet those needs.

The fourteen sessions were:

Day 1

1 Introduction to the course — short explanatory talk by one of the tutors
2 Getting to know one another — two games involving participants
3 Needs and expectations of course members — small group discussions; results were fed back to the whole group
4 *Rhymes and Reasons* — 30 minute film in which eight individuals describe their own sex education
5 Young people's needs — a structured discussion (triggered by the film) about the participants' experiences of sex education, and, following this, their understanding of young people's needs today

Day 2

6 Arguments about sex education — role-play in pairs in which turns were taken to argue on opposite points of view
7 Adolescent sexuality — quiz on adolescent sexuality and the law; used as a trigger for discussion
8 Values continuum — an exercise designed to help exploration of the range of values represented on the course; participants were asked to position themselves on a values continuum
9 Values clarification — a discussion of case studies to help clarify participants' own values; Courses 1 and 2 had an additional short exercise on language and communication about sex
10 Sexuality and contraception — quiz on factual information used to illuminate one's own attitudes.
11 Answering young people's questions — a role play/communication exercise in groups of three: one to play the role of counsellor, one a young person, one an observer; results were fed back to the whole group

Day 3

12 Courses 1 and 2: answering young people's questions — a continuation of the role play/communication exercise from Day 2. Course 3 held a discussion on participants' occupations
13 Problem-solving — a discussion method of problem-solving using

problems experienced by participants in their work situations

14 Project or practical work — planning practical methods (games, etc.) likely to be useful in participants' work situations for developing skills, etc.; presenting or trying out a particular method; reviewing presentations.

The programme was planned so that experiences in each session would contribute in some way to the attainment of the course objectives. Emphasis throughout was on 'participation', which started gradually and culminated in the project work on the afternoon of Day 3. Methods were varied and selected as examples of those participants might use in education about sexuality and personal relatinships.

The Participants' Assessment

At the end of each day participants were asked to rate the various sessions 'very worthwhile' to 'not at all worthwhile' on a five-point scale. The responses are set out in Table 2, where a weighting towards the left-hand side indicates sessions thought to have been worthwhile, while a weighting towards the right-hand side indicates the opposite.

Although there is a pronounced weighting towards the left for all the sessions, preferences clearly emerge for (14) Project work (twenty-two), (12) Discussion (twelve — Course 3 only), (7) Quiz about adolescent sexuality and the law (twenty), closely followed by (2) Getting to know one another (eighteen), (3) Young people's needs (eighteen) and (13) Problem-solving (fifteen). The session discussion (Course 3 only) relates to a particular ad hoc activity arranged by the tutors in response to the wishes of the participants. It was rated very worthwhile by twelve of the thirteen respondents. There was little indication that any of the sessions were thought to be 'not at all worthwhile'. On the other hand, there was some doubt over how worthwhile a few of the sessions were, including (1) Introduction and (9) Values clarification, about which participants' comments are set out below:

Introduction — It is important to note that (i) participants (ten) who expressed doubts about the value of this session did so mainly on the grounds that the time devoted to it was either too short or too long (rendering it slow moving); (ii) those expressing doubts were in a minority: sixteen out of thirty regarded the session as worthwhile or very worthwhile.

Values clarification — Twelve participants expressed doubts about the value of this session. Most did so on the grounds that (i) the time allowed was either too short to achieve the objectives (Course 1) or too long and getting sidetracked (Courses 2 and 3); (ii) the group was too big (Course 3 only); (iii) there was a tendency to become preoccupied with school issues (Course 3); (iv) too much polarization of professional

Table 2. The Value of Sessions 1—14

			Absent	No response	Five-point scale Very worthwhile				Not at all worthwhile
Day 1	1 Introduction	Course 1		2	5	1	3	0	1
		2			2	3	3	1	0
		3	3	1	3	2	4	1	1
		All	3	3	10	6	10	2	2
	2 Getting to know one another	Course 1		1	7	2	2	0	0
		2			4	1	2	2	0
		3	3	1	7	1	2	1	0
		All	3	2	18	4	6	3	0
	3 Needs and expectations	Course 1	1		3	7	1	0	0
		2			4	3	2	0	0
		3	3	2	6	2	1	1	0
		All	4	2	13	12	4	1	0
	4 Rhymes and reasons	Course 1	1		2	7	2	0	0
		2			4	3	2	0	0
		3	2	1	4	5	3	0	0
		All	3	1	10	15	7	0	0
	5 Young people's needs	Course 1	1		6	4	1	0	0
		2			6	1	2	0	0
		3	2	1	6	4	2	0	0
		All	3	1	18	9	5	0	0
Day 2	6 Arguments about sex	course 1	2		2	6	2	0	0
		2	1		3	3	1	1	0
		3	2	1	6	4	2	0	0
		All	5	1	11	13	5	1	0
	7 Quiz about adolescent sexuality and the law	Course 1	2		7	3	0	0	0
		2			7	1	1	0	0
		3	2	1	6	5	1	0	0
		All	4	1	20	9	2	0	0
	8 Values continuum	Course 1	2	1	1	6	2	0	0
		2			5	1	3	0	0
		3	2	1	7	3	1	1	0
		All	4	2	13	10	6	1	0
	9 Values clarification	Course 1		1	5	4	2	0	0
		2			3	1	3	0	2
		3	2		2	3	7	1	0
		All	2	1	10	8	12	1	2
	10 Quiz about contraception and sexuality	Course 1		1	4	4	3	0	0
		2			6	3	0	0	0
		3	1	1	3	6	2	1	1
		All	1	2	13	13	5	1	1
	11 Answering young people's questions I	Course 1		2	3	4	1	1	1
		2			3	4	1	0	1
		3	1	1	5	6	1	1	0
		All	1	3	11	14	3	2	2
Day 3	12 Answering young people's questions II (Courses 1 and 2 only) Discussion (Course 3 only)	Course 1	3		2	7	0	0	0
		2			2	6	0	1	0
		3	1	1	12	1	0	0	0
		All	4	1	—	—	—	—	—
	13 Problem-solving	Course 1	2		5	4	0	1	0
		2			2	6	1	0	0
		3	1		8	6	0	0	0
		All	3		15	16	1	1	0
	14 Project work	Course 1	2	1	7	2	0	0	0
		2			5	4	0	0	0
		3	1		10	3	0	1	0
		All	3	1	22	9	0	1	0

stances was allowed to developed (Course 3); (v) participants would have liked the opportunity to discuss a greater number of case studies (Course 2). Values clarification via case studies was approved by the majority as a method of approach.

The Views of Different Occupational Groups of the Particular Value of New Knowledge/Methods/Exercises Experienced on the Course

Participants were asked after the course to comment on any exercise/methods/new knowledge that they felt would be of particular value to them in their work with young people. Very few participants commented on the particular value of 'new knowledge'. The majority referred to the value of the methods and exercises used. All occupational groups reported positively that they would be willing to apply such methods in their work situation, although there were reservations from certain participants (e.g., health visitor, school nurse, EWO) on the grounds of the limited opportunities available. Some participants (e.g., social worker, school nurse, doctor) would have preferred more methods appropriate to a one-to-one situation.

Methods/exercises mentioned specifically were role-play, project work, quiz, problem-solving, values continuum and arguing from a given point of view as in arguments about sex education (another type of role-play). Of particular value were:

1　role-play (particularly in Courses 1 and 2): several participants commented that the course had positively changed their attitude to role-play, that they could now appreciate its value.
2　project work, possibly as this could be seen to be directly applicable to their work situation.

Typical comments were:

Course 1

Teacher:　　　　　　I learnt a lot more about young people through the role-play exercises. This sort of thing can be adapted and used with people to get to know each other. Also some of the project work brought new ideas and approaches to my mind in working with young people on sex education and personal relationships.

Health Visitor:　　　As I do not work with young people in a teaching capacity, I think perhaps the counselling methods I gained from others during the role-play exercises were most useful.

Course 2

School Nurse: If I can have access to the teenagers in groups, the lessons/tips learnt in managing that group will be invaluable.

EWO: The use of role-play gave me a greater insight into the feelings of both client and counsellor, and also that it is a useful method with young people.

Teacher: Reinforced the value of role-play. Made me consider using quizzes as a means of giving information. Given me a new approach to problem-solving.

Course 3

Teacher: Group work devising projects gave me some ideas for new approaches.

Intermediate
Treatment Officer: New games etc. that were introduced were very useful, and the role-plays on the last day (project work) were very valuable. Setting up the projects was an ideal manner in which to get us all thinking and putting our ideas to practice.

School Nurse: I thought the teaching and discussion methods were very useful and would apply to teaching other subjects besides sex education.

The Participants' Enjoyment of the Course

Before the course began nine participants expressed apprehension about joining in the activities on the course. Concern seemed to centre on the demands of role-play. However, the great majority stated at the end the course that they had enjoyed the three days. Their level of enjoyment on all three courses increased day by day, with Day 3 being the most relaxing and enjoyable. Where reservations were expressed these were usually in connection with certain sessions where the gain to participants was not apparent, or sessions that for them had lasted too long so that they became bored. The length of day was also criticized, as was the starting time on the first day at the end of a day's work.

Table 3. Participants' Assessment of the Attainment of Main Objectives

		Course	No response	Yes definitely		Unsure		No definitely
1	(a) To acquire some facts about sexuality	Course 1	1	5	3	2	1	0
		2	2	4	2	1	0	0
		3	3	2	6	3	1	0
		All	6	11	11	6	2	0
	(b) To be aware of relevant sources for more information	Course 1	1	4	5	2	0	0
		2	2	3	3	1	0	0
		3	3	5	4	2	1	0
		All	6	12	12	5	1	0
2	To identify feelings, attitudes, and values about sexuality of self and others	Course 1	1	4	5	2	0	0
		2	2	3	1	3	0	0
		3	3	2	5	5	0	0
		All	6	9	11	10	0	0
3	To appreciate the feelings, attitudes and values that others might have towards sexuality	Course 1	1	5	4	2	0	0
		2	2	3	3	1	0	0
		3	3	3	7	2	0	0
		All	6	11	14	5	0	0
4	To be more aware of the needs of young people with regard to sex education	Course 1	1	6	1	3	1	0
		2	2	3	3	1	0	0
		3	3	3	4	4	1	0
		All	6	12	8	8	2	0
5	To gain insight into the areas of sexuality and sex education covered by other professions/agencies and to be more aware of their approaches, values and methods	Course 1	1	5	3	2	1	0
		2	2	5	1	1	0	0
		3	3	8	3	1	0	0
		All	6	18	7	4	1	0
6	To feel willing to cooperate with and give mutual support to other agencies in work with young people in sex education	Course 1	1	7	1	3	0	0
		2	2	7	0	0	0	0
		3	3	8	1	3	0	0
		All	6	22	2	6	0	0

Attainment of the Main Objectives: The Participants' Assessment

Table 3 summarizes participants' assessment of the courses.

1   To acquire some facts about sexuality and to be aware of relevant sources for more information: Courses 1, 2, 3 — positive.

2   To identify feelings, attitudes and values about sexuality of self and others: Courses 1, 2, 3 — positive.

Although the majority of participants felt this objective had been attained there was sufficient undercurrent of uncertainty among the minority to suggest that in its present form it is too ambitious an objective for a short course. Perhaps it might be more appropriately re-worded: 'To begin to identify ...'

3   To appreciate the feelings, attitudes and values that others might have towards sexuality: Courses 1, 2, 3 — positive.

The majority of participants felt this objective had been attained, although slightly more 'with reservation' than 'without'. In addition, the uncertainty of a very small minority suggests some difficulty in attaining this objective, but not to the extent of objective 2 above.

4　To be more aware of the needs of young people with regard to sex education: Courses 1, 2, 3 — positive.

The majority of participants felt that this objective had been attained. However, the high proportion who expressed 'some reservations' along with a similar proportion 'unsure' and two 'no, with reservations' suggests that this objective was not attained to the extent to which the organizers hoped. Furthermore, the fact that it was the most important objective identified by participants before the course accentuates the need to examine how it might be more wholly attained.

5　To gain insight into the areas of sexuality and sex education covered by other professions/agencies and to be more aware of their approaches, values and methods: Courses 1, 2, 3 — positive.

The majority of participants felt that this objective had been attained. There are, however, more interesting features. In view of the innovative nature of the multiprofessional composition and the difficulty of communicating at least five different sets of professional views in very limited time, this objective might reasonably have been expected to fail. Not only did it succeed, but the positive comments of the different professionals leave no doubt that they considered the objective very important, and, evidently, much more important than they did before the course commenced (when it came fifth out of the eight objectives). Furthermore, the weight of comment directed positively at interprofessional understanding both in these comments and in the follow-up meetings underlines the fact that this aspect of the course was increasingly viewed in a more favourable light. On the negative side, there seemed to be insufficient time and opportunity for a thoroughgoing study of each other's roles and tasks as demonstrated by Course 3 making independent compensatory provision on Day 3. Courses 1 and 2 had no such provision.

6　To feel willing to cooperate with and give mutual support to other professions/agencies in work with young people in sex education: Courses 1, 2, 3 — positive.

The majority of participants felt that this objective had been attained, a view that was reinforced by the positive comments of the different professional groups. Reservations centred on the short time available for discussing *how* closer cooperation and mutual support could be brought about.

Overall, Courses 1, 2, 3 can be seen to have attained the main objectives set by the organizers, on the basis of the participants' assessment. Of particular interest are the very positive ratings of objectives 5 and 6, both concerned with interprofessional understanding and support, and more positive in emphasis than any of the other objectives, indicating a major shift from the order of priorities expressed before the course.

Post-Course Skills

A course can be attested successful in that it is seen to attain agreed objectives within a given time-span. However, when a course intends to develop skills to be applied in work situation beyond the period of the course, the measure of success experienced will not be entirely due to the influence of the course, but to a wide variety of factors external to the course, particularly those encountered in the work context of the individual course member. It was important, therefore, to determine not only immediately after the course but also several months after the extent to which participants felt an increased ability in the following skills:

1 communicating about sexuality and personal relationships;
2 developing discussion with pupils/clients/young people on their attitudes and feelings about sexuality and personal relationships.

Immediately after the course, skills 1 and 2: Courses 1, 2, 3 — positive; several months after the course: skills 1 and 2: Courses 1, 2, 3 — inconclusive. (See section on Follow-Up Meetings.)

Although immediately after the course a majority felt that they were more able to communicate about sexuality and personal relationships and to develop discussion, a high proportion of these expressed some reservations and a further one-quarter were unsure. In the very limited opportunities provided on the course to experiment with newly acquired skills these results were not unexpected. The close coincidence of the views of participants vis-à-vis both skills seemed to confirm a common lack of confidence at the time. Several months later the results at the follow-up meeting were inconclusive because the data were not available: less than half the original participants attended and therefore a full and up-to-date assessment was impossible. Nevertheless, those who did attend emphasized their greater confidence in communicating about sexuality and developing discussion and other participative activities. Overall, however, there was a strong wish for further opportunities of developing and practising communication and counselling skills.

Participants' Understanding of Each Other's Work

Participants were asked before and immediately after the course how clear they were about the nature of the work of the following occupational groups (present on the course) in the area of sex education of the young: teacher, school matron, school nurse, health visitor, social worker, doctor, education welfare officer. Courses 1, 2, 3 — positive.

While generally participants were of the view that there had been an increase in understanding about the nature of each other's work, the imbalances in each of the three courses (referred to under Recruitment) clearly reduced learning opportunities. On the other hand, where an occupational group was represented in all three courses, e.g., the teachers, health visitors and education welfare officers, the overall 'increase in clarity' was very high. Course 3 with its specially arranged discussion on the participants' occupations showed above-average increases.

Follow-Up Meetings

These were two follow-up meetings arranged several months after the end of the courses to give former participants an opportunity to critically appraise the courses and to report on any effect the courses may have had on their subsequent work. Attendance was low: less than half, although a number of non-attenders sent messages of regret. Since overall there were six occupational groups represented and former members of all three courses, it was felt that the comments they made could be considered to be fairly representative. Nevertheless, the meetings were denied the views of doctors and social workers who were represented on the original courses. Participants made the following comments on important features of the course:

1 *Organization* — positive:
   The venue, the FPA Centre, away from the work situation and its associated problems provided an opportunity for objective assessment of problems in a supportive atmosphere. The FPA staff provided a warm welcome and delicious lunches.
   The groups were about the right size with a fair balance of occupations. Younger participants appreciated the opportunity to discuss sexuality with older ones, an opportunity they seldom had in their work situation.
   The lead given by *the tutors* was good, carefully prepared, responsive and enthusiastic.
   — *negative:*
   Pre-course apprehension about such 'threatening' activities as role-play was experienced by several participants new to FPA courses and who did not attend the preliminary meeting (arranged before the course).

The groups were unbalanced with respect to the sexes; the male viewpoint was lacking.

The time was too short, e.g., for in-depth discussion, to explore and break down stereotypes.

The starting time on the first day at the end of a day's work meant that many arrived tired out.

Better area coordination might have resulted in a wider range and improved balance of professions/agencies.

2   *Methods — positive:*

Active participation as in role-play and 'games' exercises was much preferred to sitting and listening. The method of working in threes as opposed to performing in front of the whole group was confidence-building and non-threatening. In addition, role-play methods increased understanding, sensitivity, and depth of thought and feeling.

The *variety of methods* employed was appreciated.

The acquisition of some *counselling skills* was noted.

The recognition that everyone had a *right to an opinion* was valued.

— negative:

The acquisition of some counselling skills left participants with a feeling of how inadequately equipped they were to counsel, and a wish for this deficiency to be remedied.

Too little opportunity to practise games, etc.

3   *Interprofessional contact — positive:*

An *increase in knowledge and understanding* of other roles and areas of work and associated difficulties and problems. In addition, an opportunity to break down stereotypes of other professions.

A valuing of meeting and *sharing problems* from work with others who were supportive in an 'away from work' situation; and a knowledge of who one might contact in the future.

An opportunity for *reappraising* one's own and other's *attitudes* to sexuality and sex education.

As a result of working together for three days interprofessional *relationships* were strengthened.

Members of the *same professional group* but who work in different institutions or districts found it beneficial to compare notes.

— negative:

Too little time to break down stereotypes.

Too oriented towards *school* (one course).

A wish for the *range of professionals to be widened* to include solicitors, probation officers, police, magistrates, etc.

Too few agencies/professionals *linked with a specific school* which could have meant a greater carry-over beyond the course.

On one course a tendency for the members of one professional group to form a *clique*.

A feeling of *isolation* expressed by the sole members of a professional group.

4 *Personal outcomes of the course*

Clarification of own views and feelings; greater self-awareness.

Greater confidence in oneself and ability to communicate and present ideas.

More knowledge of sexuality and sex education to draw upon rather than 'informed guess work'.

Knowing the FPA Centre is accessible and supportive.

5 *Practical outcomes of the course related to the work situation*

There had been some *cautious experimentation* with the methods learnt on the course, e.g., role-play, games, 'arguments in pairs' and values continuum, three of them in a classroom situation. A teacher and an EWO felt confident enough to use the games but so far had not had an opportunity to organize sessions.

For professionals associated with one school a *heightened interest* in what was going on there.

The beginnings of active cooperation between different professional groups in that, for example, one teacher had since the course recognized a counselling role and skills in the school EWO and had begun to draw upon these. Another teacher had drawn on the counselling skills of one of the tutors, and was much more aware of the support that could be enlisted from other professionals locally.

6 *Future practical needs*

Future courses or meetings should continue to be held off the premises of the agencies represented.

Such courses or meetings should provide opportunities for participants to work with, as well as air grievances about, agencies present. Clearly a good facilitator would be required and from outside the agencies represented, if there were to be positive outcomes.

Two specific practical needs expressed were:

(a) *a course on counselling* to promote counselling skills and confidence in using them.

(b) *an after-care mutual support group* for the members of the different caring professions; the aims, etc. to be decided by the members. Such aims might be examining further the stereotypes that hinder mutual understanding, building up members' confidence to look at 'feelings', discovering other professionals' perspectives on and approaches to moral issues, and the ethics of sex education.

More opportunities to learn about patterns of sexual behaviour in young people and their consequences.

Ways of working through the family to help young people.

Ways of helping 'normal' families with their sexual problems.

Methods of teaching teenagers and their evaluation.

George Campbell (UK)

Tutors' Comments

Three months after the last of three courses, the impression is that the courses did meet the overall aims in helping participants feel more confident, comfortable and sensitive in working with young people in the area of sexuality and personal relationships.

As far as individual course members were concerned, there seemed to be varying levels of satisfaction with the course. This is to be expected, but there did seem to be a link between satisfaction and levels of commitment and participation. The school doctors, for example, varied considerably in their response. They had apparently been given the impression by their superiors that attendance was more or less compulsory but that they need not attend the whole course. Although the FPA usually makes it clear that participants must contract to attend the whole course, on this occasion because of the need to recruit a wide range of professions, the doctors were allowed to attend on their own terms. This proved to be a mistake as it was very clear that the two doctors who seemed to enjoy and benefit from the course were those who were keen to attend and sorry to miss sessions when circumstances forced their absence. On the other hand, the two doctors who attended only because they were expected to missed more sessions, participated less and seemed to enjoy the course less and benefit less.

The significant difference between these courses and the usual FPA courses in sexuality and personal relationships education is that these were intended to develop greater interprofessional understanding and, where possible, cooperation. This was achieved to a certain extent as participants did make contact and came to like and trust people in other professions and clearly expressed a willingness to cooperate and mutually support in the future.

However, it was noticeable that at times of tension in one group, barriers between the professions became more obvious. It would need either a longer course, or one consisting of a series of linked modules, to explore these barriers as they arise in the group. It should also be possible in a future course to programme sessions where these barriers could be explored by studying stereotypes, assumptions and anxieties in a more generalized way.

The courses were quite effective in helping participants to appreciate some of the problems and perspectives of other professions but this could probably have been organized more systematically. For example, in one course where there were two quite vocal education welfare officers, other participants seemed to learn a great deal about the EWO's work and their problems. On Course 3, however, where there was only one EWO very little seemed to be learned about his work until it was brought out in a specially planned session where the work of each agency was specifically discussed (Day 3, Session 1).

Many participants expressed the desire for continuing liaison after the course, so the course effectively met the aims of developing the willingness to cooperate and give mutual support to other professions and agencies. However, if it were possible to have a longer course, the barriers to cooperative work could be explored, interprofessional understanding and respect could be extended, the structures for mutual support could be created, and the increased skills and sensitivity of those people working in the areas of sexuality and personal relationships could be used to their full advantage.

Conclusion

A multidisciplinary course must have a certain minimum range of professional groups in order to provide cross-disciplinary perspectives. The idea of bringing together those professional groups linked with a pair of comprehensive schools was a sound one, as was the policy of securing the cooperation of senior officers to help bring this about. What was achieved was a very satisfactory range, although understandably, particular gaps caused some disappointment and frustration to participants.

The overall aim of the course was complex but, nevertheless, in the view of participants wholly achieved. The difficulties encountered by participants and evaluators in coming to terms with the term 'being comfortable' suggests that this part of the aim be revised, perhaps by using 'self-aware' in its place.

The overall value of the course was considered high by most participants, some of whom had started off with already high expectations.

The main objectives were *all* attained, the most positively being the last two which were both concerned with interprofessional aspects. This is of particular interest as it represents a marked shift in the professional orientation of participants, compared with before the course. On the other hand, the reservations and uncertainties of minorities are pointers to some revision either of objectives or course format. A course with so much to offer might gain significantly were it to concentrate on three key conditions:

1   the creation of more time to enable participants to develop further their knowledge, ideas, attitudes and skills either by a longer course or a two-module course. The latter would have the double advantage of being less tiring and of providing an opportunity for an intermodule practical task stemming from work in the first module;
2   to continue to work towards a recruitment policy based on the catchments of a group of schools, conducted with the cooperation of the officials of the various services, with as representative a range of professions/agencies as practicable, but inclusive of general practitioners, social workers, police and probation officers;
3   to include at least one session specifically concerned with defining the roles and tasks of the different professions/agencies.

If courses were to be conducted observing these conditions and followed up by the establishment of the kind of mutual support group requested by several participants during the course, and enlarged upon by those at the follow-up meetings, this could be the start of a local community self-help group able to initiate, monitor and provide for their own professional development with the minimum of outside help.

The Family Planning Association is to be congratulated upon taking the initiative in such an important and yet difficult area, and not least making public the results of an independent assessment of its work.

Reference

1 CAMPBELL, G. and GRAY, G. (1982) *Course Evaluation: An Introduction to Sexuality and Personal Relationships Education*, series of three multidisciplinary courses conducted in Basingstoke in November 1981 and February 1982, Family Planning Association and Department of Education, University of Southampton. This report sets out in greater detail the planning, organization, conduct and evaluation of the three courses upon which this chapter is based.

Part 5. Cooperative Health Education in the United Kingdom: Case Studies

Introduction

The purpose of Part 5 is to sample recent progress in one country, the United Kingdom, at national, regional and local levels. The host country is the obvious choice, not because progress is more marked there but because information on developments is more accessible due to many of the individuals concerned being in close and regular contact through meetings, conferences and joint tasks.

While developments in school health education in the UK may appear to be impressive, there is still much to be done, since only about half of the local education authorities are fully committed to the national Schools Health Education Project and an even smaller proportion of the nation's schools. At government level there is no declared national policy on school health education such as exists in The Netherlands. At regional level few regional health authorities have demonstrated a clear and ongoing commitment to the place of health education in policies of health promotion. At local level school-community cooperation is very patchy, with the majority of positively evaluated experiments depending more upon the efforts of local enthusiasts and entrepreneurs than on any more widely-based long-term plan. Progress however is being made at all levels, with the support of national organizations such as the Health Education Council, regional organizations such as the Wessex Regional Health Authority and about fifty local education authorities and many other local organizations. What follows is merely a selection of some recent work, but work which is firmly grounded and moving confidently in an upwards direction in spite of the obstacles.

Innovation and Dissemination at National Level: The Role of the Health Education Council

Donald Reid

What is the role of a government-funded education organization in a country with the most decentralized school system in the world? Finding the answer has been the task of the Health Education Council for England, Wales and Northern Ireland (HEC) since it commenced support for school health education in 1972. The HEC is a nominally independent organization wholly financed by the British Government through its Department of Health and Social Security. With a current annual budget of about £9 million, the HEC's functions include:

1   the conduct of programmes and mass campaigns of health education 'within the framework of government policy' and in cooperation with local health, education and other authorities, voluntary bodies etc.;
2   the provision of training for health educators and other professionals involved in health education;
3   the production of over 20 million free posters and leaflets annually, many of which are used by schools;
4   the conduct of research and evaluation especially relating to HEC programmes.

School Health Education and the HEC: Where to Begin?

In 1972 the Council faced the task of deciding how best to promote school health education with the limited resources at its disposal. On reviewing the existing provision in British schools it was obvious that basic information on health was readily available to teachers from a variety of sources — including the HEC's own leaflets. However, teaching methods in this field had progressed little beyond traditional fact-giving, didactic presentations. Typically the learner was not actively involved in the lesson and little attention was given to the many psycho-social factors involved in making personal decisions about health. In addition, there was no consensus about the place of health education in the curriculum. In some schools, e.g. middle schools in Leeds, it was taught exclusively by health workers and not by teachers. Others saw it as a separate subject to be taught only by specialist teachers, although a growing number saw it as a task to be shared by the entire staff.

The HEC therefore identified two priorities for action at this time:

1 supporting the development of active, non-didactic teaching methods which emphasized discussion of attitudes, values and feelings;
2 promoting debate about the position of health education in the curriculum, with the aim of achieving consensus.

Accordingly, the Council's first initiative for schools was to set up the HEC 'Living Well' project,[1] directed by Peter McPhail at Cambridge University. Between 1972 and 1976 McPhail's team produced a series of stimulus materials with teachers' guides, to promote non-didactic methods in health education.

At about this time also, support for school health education was being considered by the Schools Council (SC), an organization similar to the HEC but funded by the government Department of Education and Science and by local education authorities, with responsibility for the entire curriculum. In 1973 the SC set up a three-year project to examine the place of health education in primary schools and simultaneously to promote the use of non-didactic methods. The HEC accordingly joined with the SC (and other sponsors) to fund this major development. The project, later known as the Schools Council/HEC Project Health Education 5–13[2], produced two substantial teachers' guides for the 5–8 and 9–13 age ranges under Trefor Williams' direction at Colchester Institute of Higher Education. A jointly funded extension of the project for slow learners (5–16) was produced in 1983.[3]

To help define the place of health education in secondary schools, the two Councils again combined in 1976 to set up a working party on organization and methods. This group had little difficulty in reaching a consensus in its report,[4] along these lines:

1 schools should be urged to draw up policies for health education and social education, to be coordinated by a senior member of staff;
2 a core course comprising health and social education, with education for personal relationships, should be provided for all;
3 major contributions, appropriately coordinated within the overall policy, were also needed from the various specialist subjects (e.g. biology, home economics);
4 health education as a specialist subject in its own right, leading to an

examination at age sixteen, was not recommended, since it would inevitably come to be seen as an option for the less able.

To implement the working paper's findings, a second major joint project (SC/HEC 13–18) was set up in 1977[5] again led by Trefor Williams, first at Colchester and later at the Department of Education, University of Southampton. In addition to materials designed to stimulate non-didactic approaches, as before, major emphasis was given to the development of a training manual. This was intended to assist schools in defining the role of the coordinator and the contributions of each specialist subject.

As a result of these and other initiatives, by the early 1980s health education had become firmly identified with the wider field of personal and social education, including moral, political and careers education. To help define the place of health education within this growing area, the HEC in 1981 invited the Schools Council to commission a major report on personal and social education.[6] This helped further to emphasize the need for broadly defined core courses and for appropriate training in this important but difficult field.

Training and Dissemination

The importance of training and dissemination generally had in fact been evident since 1977. Publication of the first two major school projects (5–13) and 'Living Well') with the Secondary School Organization Report led to considerable discussion about the implementation of their findings. Producing new materials or agreeing a set of recommendations is a relatively easy task compared to the problem of persuading 500,000 teachers in Britain to implement them. The difficulty is even greater if 499,900 have had no direct involvement in their creation. It became clear, then, that a major investment in dissemination was required if the new approaches were to be widely adopted.

The experience gained at the time and later led to the formulation of the following principles for successful dissemination of HEC schools projects:

1 Dissemination must be given serious consideration before any new activity commences. Even before major national funding is granted, prior evidence that an innovation is likely to be practicable at local level is essential.

2 In addition, acceptability to a wide audience of dissemination 'agents', such as health education officers and local education authority (LEA) staff, should be tested at an early stage, preferably through an initial conference. Essentially, in commercial terms, this involves establishing the 'marketability' of the innovation.

3 Development teams, once set up, must work in close cooperation with a network of trial schools, from the outset.

4   Following a development phase, provision must be made for a dissemination phase. This will require a central team at least as large as the original development team. Their functions will include the production of training manuals, videos, etc., and the conduct of courses organized to train teams of trainers in each district — rather than training individual teachers.

5   Local training teams should also be encouraged to train 'institutions' rather than individual teachers. This means training several teachers from each of a few schools, rather than one teacher from many schools. In the long run, concentration in a few schools is the more effective method. It is also essential to involve the headteacher in each case, at least at the outset.

6   Every effort should be made to encourage local groups to amend schemes to suit their own needs, so that new ideas come to be 'their property'.[7]

7   Finally, it must be accepted that the whole process, from the first consideration of a new idea to its adoption by a substantial number of teachers, may take up to ten years. The cost of dissemination will probably exceed the cost of the initial development phase.

Dissemination in Practice

Adherence to these principles has led to a selective approach to development, sometimes resulting in rejection of apparently promising proposals. For example, the HEC unlike several other international organizations in Europe , has not supported British trials of the Californian CLASP project.[8] This well researched scheme involves the use of 16-year-olds to teach 12-year-olds 'how to resist peer pressures' to smoke, drink and take drugs. Despite the considerable evidence for the success of this technique in health terms, it was considered by HEC to be too impracticable for use in British schools. The wisdom of this decision has since been confirmed by its original Californian developers, who have been compelled to modify the scheme considerably.

The importance of demonstrating acceptability at local level before commencing national development has been shown by the success of two more recent HEC-funded projects, Active Tutorial Work (ATW) and the 'My Body' project.

ATW was originally developed by Jill Baldwin and colleagues in Lancashire[9] to provide a structured course of personal and social education for use during tutor (or form teacher) lessons. Its success within Lancashire as a vehicle for the introduction of non-didactic methods led HEC to hold a national conference for LEA advisers in 1979 devoted to the ATW project. Their enthusiastic welcome led the Council to set up a national team, led by Jill Baldwin and Andy Smith, to provide training throughout Britain.

Sixty-three LEAs (out of a total of 109) had taken part in the scheme by 1983, and requests for the team's services greatly exceeded their capacity to provide training.

A similar lengthy period of local trials preceded the national development of the HEC 'My Body' project,[10] an activity-based project for 10–12-year-olds with special emphasis on smoking. Five years of 'grass-roots' experience in Sheffield under Pat Elkington's leadership, preceded three years of national development directed by John Gaskin and a further three years' dissemination under Dave McLeavy. The result has been universal acclaim with over thirty LEAs involved in the training programme within months of publication in 1983. As many teachers have said of the project's publications: 'You can tell they were written by practising teachers.'

Five years' labour in Cambridgeshire and neighbouring LEAs were necessary also for the HEC Dental Health Study led by Michael Craft and Ray Crouchell to produce the international prize winning 'Natural Nashers' project.[11] 'Natural Nashers', a three-lesson course on dental hygiene for 13–14-year-olds is now, however, the subject of a major dissemination programme in over twenty areas.

ATW, 'My Body' and 'Natural Nashers' are all examples of the most important task undertaken by any national body in this field — to facilitate the rapid dissemination of good practice nationally. This approach is often referred to as a 'periphery-periphery' model of dissemination, as opposed to a 'centre-periphery' model, where ideas are disseminated 'downwards' from a central team. 'Centre-periphery' innovations, though less likely to be as successful as 'periphery-periphery', can nevertheless make a noticeable impact if the principles of successful dissemination are observed. For example, a major reason for the success of the 5–13 and 13–18 projects has been the insistence of Trefor Williams upon working closely with a wide network of trial schools from the outset. While this inevitably leads to delay, and endless and expensive travel for project teams, the result is a project with considerably improved prospects for widespread adoption.

Finally, successful implementation invariably depends heavily on training. This has resulted in the HEC funding the development of sophisticated training manuals (e.g., the 5–13, 13–18, and 'My Body' projects); and training videos (e.g., 5–13, 'Natural Nashers' and 'My Body'). HEC grants to participating LEAs to cover the costs of releasing teachers for training have also been made available for the 'Natural Nashers' and 'My Body' projects.

Evaluation

From the outset the HEC has accepted the need to give high priority to evaluation. Two kinds of evaluation, formative and summative, have been

undertaken. Formative evaluation has been conducted to assess the acceptability of projects to teachers, pupils (and even parents). Following the
Schools Councils pattern, evaluation of this type has been routinely
conducted by evaluators attached to all the major projects. Information
gathered in this way has led to numerous improvements in the design of
materials as the work has proceeded. Summative evaluation to assess the
effects of projects in their final form has also been carried out in respect of
certain developments. As a matter of policy, summative evaluation has
generally only been conducted when projects have undergone modifications
through use by classroom teachers remote from the original developers.

Unlike some international organizations, the HEC has generally re-
sisted the temptation to evaluate the first drafts of new schemes still in the
hands of their enthusiastic initiators, and perhaps taught personally by them
in their own schools; 'success' under these circumstances, is usually assured.
Typical results of HEC evaluation have included these findings:

1   The HEC 'My Body' project has been found to have favourable
    effects on knowledge and attitudes to smoking among pupils;[12] has
    some influence on parents' smoking[13] and is believed to halve the
    rate of experimental smoking among pupils for up to two years
    later;[14]
2   The 'Natural Nashers' project also achieves significant gains in
    knowledge and attitudes, especially relating to willingness to take
    personal responsibility for oral hygiene. More important still, it
    leads to definite reductions in teenage plaque scores.[15]

Summing Up: What Has HEC Achieved?

The precise value of all of these innovations, schemes, evaluations and
developments in terms of either health or education cannot be readily
measured. Perhaps the anecdotal evidence about truancy reduction from
'My Body' project schools ('he only comes when we're doing the project') is
the strongest single recommendation from an educational point of view. The
gains to the nation's health may take decades to materialize.

However, in terms of dissemination of ideas, the transformation of
school health education between 1973 and 1983 is evident from a wealth of
statistics, e.g.:

1   In 1973 school coordinators for health education were almost
    non-existent. By 1983, up to half all secondary schools had a
    designated coordinator.
2   In 1981, after years of apparent disinterest, the Department of
    Education and Science (DES) firmly recommended the inclusion of
    health education as part of the 'core curriculum' for every pupil;[16]

and at about this time DES inspectors began to include health education in formal inspections.

3 The SC/HEC 5–13 project is in substantial use in at least 5000 schools, with another 5000 or more making 'some use' of the project or its associated TV programmes.

4 The SC/HEC 13–18 project was already in use in 700 schools (15 per cent of the total) involving 56,000 pupils, prior to publication in 1982.

5 Sixty-three LEAs have taken part in ATW training, fifty in training for 13–18, and virtually all of the 109 LEAs in the HEC's territory have taken part in training in the use of one or more of HEC's sponsored projects.

6 The HEC spends about £2 million annually on schools, and the National Health Service, through local health education officers, contributes perhaps a further £3 million. But as a result of the growing partnership between education and health, LEAs spend at least £200 million annually on health education (based on 0.6 of a teacher per school). In this way every penny of NHS investment is now multiplied forty times, and the return is likely to grow still larger in the years to come.

Not surprisingly credit for these major advances must be broadly spread. Although the purpose of this chapter is to describe HEC's involvement, the contributions of other national bodies, project teams, LEAs, District Health Authorities, and individual advisers, HEOs and teachers greatly exceed HEC's in sheer volume. But, along with the Schools Council (as it then was), the HEC can fairly claim a pivotal role as catalyst and facilitator.

The Future

Despite the long litany of improving statistics, much remains to be done. All the successful major projects require continuing support for dissemination, and regular updating of materials. But increasing emphasis can be expected in future on methods of integrating health and education. For example, teaching about rubella just before vaccinations are offered is known to increase the subsequent uptake of vaccinations[17] but how many schools time their teaching accordingly? Green and his colleagues have provided a conceptual framework for schools, in this field;[18] they suggest analyzing health problems in terms of all the factors which predispose towards, reinforce or maintain 'potentially hazardous behaviours'. For maximum contribution to health, schools can then try to plan their teaching in cooperation with outside agencies as necessary, and taking account also of other influences. Two examples of success in reducing unintended teenage pregnancies in Swedish and US schools have both involved cooperation between family planning clinic workers and schools, in addition to intensive sex education courses.[19,20] Similarly, if schools seriously wish to reduce teenage smoking they need to consider:[21]:

1 providing basic facts;
2 teaching resistance to peer pressures, advertizing, etc.;
3 developing an overall school policy for smoking (e.g. teacher smoking);
4 asking parents to discuss the hazards of smoking with their children;
5 conducting prevalence studies, both to determine the key age groups for education and to measure their own success;
6 reminding local tobacconists that sales to under-16s are illegal.

Assistance with most of these tasks is, or shortly will be, available from the HEC, as a variety of publications and teachers' guides are completed. Over 150 schools have already used the HEC-funded health behaviour research questionnaires developed by John Balding at Exeter University to investigate pupil self-reported health behaviour, covering a wide variety of topics.[22] Several schools are known to have adjusted their curriculum as a result.

Lack of space prevents mention of many other HEC-funded developments relating to physical fitness, solvent abuse, alcohol education, science teaching, pre-service teacher training, and a variety of special projects for the 16–19 age range. Education for parenthood, also, has become a major focus of interest following the setting up of joint projects with the Open University and with UNICEF. An encyclopaedic description of every one of HEC's current twenty-five projects for schools is, however, unnecessary for the purpose of this chapter, which is to examine the influence of a national organization on the teaching of health education in one country. How far the HEC has succeeded in this field is for others to judge. (*The opinions expressed in this article are those of the author alone and not necessarily those of the Health Education Council.*)

Notes

1 HEALTH EDUCATION COUNCIL (1977) *'Living Well' Project*, Cambridge, Cambridge University Press (out of print).
2 SCHOOLS COUNCIL/HEALTH EDUCATION COUNCIL PROJECT (1977) *Health Education 5–13*, London, T. Nelson and Sons.
3 SCHOOLS COUNCIL/HEALTH EDUCATION COUNCIL PROJECT (1983) *Health Education 5–13 — Extension for Slow Learners ('Fit for Life')* London, Macmillan Education.
4 SCHOOLS COUNCIL (1976) *Health Education in Secondary Schools* Schools Council Working Paper 57, in conjunction with the HEC, London, Evans/Methuen Educational.
5 SCHOOLS COUNCIL/HEALTH EDUCATION COUNCIL PROJECT (1982) *Health Education 13–18*, London, Forbes Publications.

6 DAVID, K. (1982) *Personal and Social Education in Secondary Schools* York, Longman for the Schools Council.

7 BOLAM, R. (1983) *Strategies for School Improvement* Mimeo, Paris, Organization for Economic Cooperation and Development (OECD).

8 McALISTER, A. *et al.* (1980) 'A pilot study of smoking, alcohol and drug abuse prevention', *American Journal of Public Health*, 70, pp. 719–21.

9 BALDWIN, J. and WELLS, H. (1979–82) *Active Tutorial Work, Books 1–5*, Oxford, Basil Blackwell in association with Lancashire LEA.

10 HEALTH EDUCATION COUNCIL (1983) *'My Body' Project 10–12*, London, Heinemann Education.

11 HEALTH EDUCATION COUNCIL DENTAL HEALTH STUDY (DHS) (1980) *'Natural Nashers' Project*, details from the DHS at Old Addenbrooke's Hospital, Cambridge, CB2 1QF.

12 WILCOX, B. *et al.* (1978) 'Smoking education in children: UK trials of an international project', *International Journal of Health Education* 21, 4, pp. 236–44.

13 WILCOX, B. *et al.* (1981) 'Do children influence their parents' smoking? *'Health Education Journal*, 40, 1, pp. 5–10.

14 GILLIES, P.A. and WILCOX, B. (1983) 'Reducing the risk of smoking against the young', *Public Health*, (in the press, 1983).

15 CRAFT, M., *et al.* (1981) 'Preventive dental health in adolescents ...,' *Commun, Dent. Oral Epidemiol.* 9, pp. 199–206.

16 DEPARTMENT OF EDUCATION AND SCIENCE WELSH OFFICE (1981) *The School Curriculum*, London, HMSO.

17 JONES, S.A.M. (1980) 'A control trial of health education to promote the uptake of rubella immunisation in schools', summary only in *Journal of Epidemiological and Community Medicine*, 34, pp. 151–2.

18 GREEN, L.W. *et al.* (1980) *Health Education Planning: A Diagnostic Approach*, Palo Alto, Calif., Mayfield Press.

19 REID, D.J. (1981) 'School sex education and the causes of unintended teenage pregnancies — a review', *Health Education Journal*, 41, 1, p. 4.

20 BROWN, P. (1983) 'The Swedish approach to sex education and adolescent pregnancy: Some impressions', *Family Planning Perspectives*, 15, 2, pp. 90–5.

21 REID, D.J. (1985) 'The prevention of smoking in children: A review of current (UK) developments and associated research', *Health Education Journal* 45, March 1985.

22 BALDING, J. (1983) 'Developing the Health Related Behaviour Questionnaire', *Education and Health*, 1, 1, pp. 9–13 (Journal of the HEC Schools Health Education Unit, St Luke's, University of Exeter).

Some Recent Work of Other National Organizations Involved in Health Education

George Campbell

In England, the Department of Education and Science (DES) and Her Majesty's Inspectorate (HMI) have a national responsibility for laying down curricular guidelines and assessing standards in the formal education system. In recent years (1978 and 1979) HMI have produced national surveys of primary and secondary education. In the Secondary Survey of the four aspects selected for special study, one was 'the personal and social development of the pupils and their general preparation for adult living'. Within this aspect HMI take the view that health education should be an important component of formal education whether it be 'free-standing' (existing independently) or taught as an integral part of other subjects such as human biology or home economics. However, they also draw attention to the vulnerability of health education and other aspects of personal and social education which are not always clearly identified with particular specialistic subjects. This problem becomes acute when the school's curricular philosophy is unclear, and effective curricular coordination is lacking.

HMI have specific subject committees to review the national situation, receive comments, set out guidelines and publish working papers for further discussion and comment by those in the education service. There is a Health Education Committee; in addition, the Science Committee and the Home Economics Committee both include reference to health education in their deliberations.

In recent years the DES have produced many memoranda bearing directly or indirectly on health education and circulated to all local education authorities and schools in the country, for example, on drugs misuse (1977) and more generally on the curriculum (1980). The DES also advise Parliament, and where insufficient is known about a problem causing concern will commission research. For example, the problems facing most young parents are complex and unanticipated, and there has been little preparation in the school curriculum for dealing with them. The DES therefore commissioned the University of Aston to study formal and informal education in secondary schools which would have a positive contribution to make to the social and practical skills needed in parenthood. This has involved examining the views of pupils, teachers, parents and members of the community about the purpose, content and value of this aspect of education for young people.

Two other national organizations in the UK which are making important and original contributions to the development of health education in school and community are the Teachers' Advisory Council on Alcohol and Drug Education (TACADE) and the Family Planning Association (FPA).

TACADE is organized into two units. The unit concerned with alcohol and drug education concentrates on developing training courses and teaching materials which help teachers review the area of alcohol and drug education with young people. The second unit is the Health Education Development Unit, which is concerned with the overall development of schools' health education. It concerns itself particularly with curriculum planning and organization of health education in schools, the in-service training of teachers and other health educators in health education, and researching and developing classroom and in-service methods in health education. Much of the value of TACADE derives from the close and effective links it has forged with other national organizations such as the HEC national health education projects such as SHEP and regional and local organizations such as LEAs and individual schools. Through the clear, field-tested advice and guidance it offers through its numerous publications, consultancy and information centre it has considerably advanced thinking and innovations in many schools in the complex school-community problem areas of alcohol and drug education, not to mention health education generally. One of its more recent major publications has been *Free to Choose*, a ten-unit pack of drug education material, with which are linked supporting training courses for health educators in their local areas.

The FPA, or more specifically the FPA Education Unit, has been in operation since 1972, charged with the task of educating and training professional groups in the area of personal relationships and sexuality. Since the mid-1970s Unit staff have designed and developed courses that seek to involve participants much more than formerly in their own learning process. Courses are run by a small team of FPA group leaders or tutors using participatory methods such as role-play, group discussion, quizzes and communication exercises. The scope of the work has been extended to cover the wide range of issues arising out of personal relationships and sexuality. The groups taught now include the whole range of 'caring' professions and agencies as well as many lay groups. The general objectives of the courses are:

1   to provide relevant factual information about human sexuality and relationships;

2 to increase course members' awareness of the needs of those with whom they work;
3 to increase course members' sensitivity and comfort with their own and others' sexuality;
4 to demonstrate methods of education in sexuality and personal relationships.

The aims, objectives, content and methods vary somewhat from course to course, but the general goal is to build up knowledge and to create a sensitive awareness and understanding by participants of their own attitudes and other people's in such a way that they can increase their competence and confidence in the handling of sex education and personal relationships issues with their client groups. The courses are designed to work in two ways, so that they are relevant both to course members themselves and to course members in relation to their work.

The FPA does not present its approach as the total solution. Instead it hopes that the experience of the course will enable participants to improve and develop their own strategies and skills alongside others who attend the course and then in their own work setting. Regular courses in personal relationships and sexuality are held in London and the regions for multidisciplinary groups, youth and community workers, teachers, health education officers and other professional groups. The Unit also designs 'made-to-measure' courses to meet the needs of a particular organization, e.g., social service department, health authority, education authority, youth service, nursing staff of a hospital, residential staff.

Within the UK Scotland organizes and administers its own educational system and therefore has its own advisory body for health education: the Scottish Health Education Group (SHEG). Although the responsibility of SHEG is for health education in Scotland and it is therefore independent of national organizations in England, there is close liaison between the two countries to the extent that some initiatives which are manifestly of benefit to both countries are jointly funded. The Schools Health Education Project (SHEP) with a Scottish Regional Coordinator is a case in point. Much of the work of SHEG is concerned with the organization of compaigns, sometimes multimedia in scope, to increase community awareness and understanding of health issues. It also produces publications and materials, and promotes research. In principle, there are five strands to SHEG's activities:

1 helping to determine priorities in health education for Scotland;
2 designing programmes to meet these priorities;
3 conducting research in health education and evaluating its own programmes at national level;
4 helping all groups and organizations with their own health education programmes;
5 encouraging people working in the wide range of professional and voluntary organizations to develop their skills in health education.

Although the Republic of Ireland lies outside the UK, informal links between the two countries are close in the field of health education. The Health Education Bureau (HEB) was established by the Irish Government in 1975 and has gradually expanded its role and influence. The Education and Training Division is responsible for the initiation, development and implementation of health education programmes in schools. Much of its work is assisted by the Bureau's policy of collaboration with other national and regional organizations in identifying key areas of research, contributing to their funding and disseminating the findings via *HEB News*, conferences and training courses. One recent example is the 1981 survey of post-primary schools in the city and county of Dublin to determine the extent to which drugs were being used by children. This was a project organized jointly by HEB, the Medico-Social Research Board, the Irish Cancer Society and the Department of Community Health, Trinity College, Dublin. Its findings are fully reported and discussed in *HEB News* (1983). An earlier issue of *HEB News* took as its theme the creation of a diversity of links between school and community.

No survey of health education would be complete without reference to those national institutions of higher education which have developed the study of the subject to an advanced level. In addition to various centres of research into health education, several institutions have developed taught courses to diploma and master's levels. To take England as an example, no fewer than seven institutions of higher education offer advanced courses in health education: Bristol Polytechnic, Leeds Polytechnic and London Polytechnic of the South Bank offer diploma courses; the University of London at Chelsea College and the Institute of Education, the University of Manchester and the University of Southampton offer master's degree courses. All of these institutions have been assisted in developing their courses by funding from the Health Education Council. Since a number of them have also set up research projects funded by the HEC it is evident that much of the impetus for high-level research, as well as the training of personnel, derives directly from HEC policies. The encouragement given by HEC to those involved in teaching and research to meet regularly to review progress and coordinate efforts is also an important factor in establishing an overall national picture which can then be critically examined. Those involved in the teaching of advanced courses meet together at least once each year, while those involved in research and development projects meet together every two years for a five-day conference. In fact, were it not for the positive intervention of HEC, it is doubtful if health education would feature significantly in higher education in England.

Achieving Interprofessional Cooperation at Regional Level in Wessex

George Campbell and Donald Nutbeam

In the UK there are regional health authorities (RHAs) but no regional education authorities. On the other hand, there are local education authorities (LEAs) which in area or population terms are large, and some not much smaller than some of the RHAs, which can give a misleading impression when the terms 'local' and 'regional' are used. To complicate the picture further, sub-divisions of LEAs are known as 'areas' and correspond approximately to the RHA sub-divisions which are termed 'districts'. Since RHAs and LEAs rarely have boundaries which coincide, the achievement of any degree of cooperation between the two main bodies concerned with health education becomes difficult even if the will is there.

Difficulties, however, can be overcome. Centres of higher education, especially universities, where they have retained close teacher in-service education links with the LEAs of their former regional training divisions, may be in a strong position to promote cooperation at regional level with RHAs. Such cooperation could be facilitated by a university by virtue of its political independence, but clearly only if it had a strong and definable commitment to health education and its credibility rating was high in the eyes of the RHA and LEAs.

The University of Southampton, as one centre of health education in the UK, has strong links with the LEAs in its region and has provided the foundation for such a development in the Wessex Region of central-southern England. This feature has been matched by the Wessex RHA which is almost unique in the UK in having a Positive Health Team: a strong multidisciplinary advisory team concerned with health education and health promotion across the region. The key tasks of the Wessex Positive Health Team are to monitor health status, commission research and advise the RHA on policies, strategies and methods of health promotion.

In February 1982, in cooperation with the University of Southampton Department of Community Medicine, the Wessex RHA Positive Health Team held a conference entitled 'Prospects for Prevention in Wessex'.[1] The primary aim of the conference was to enable the newly constituted District Health Authorities (DHAs) to identify in advance the many challenges and future opportunities for health promotion in the health service.

In addition to links between the University Department of Community Medicine and the RHA, the Department of Education, in pursuing a positive regional policy of in-service education with its five LEA partners — Dorset, Hampshire, Isle of Wight, West Sussex and Wiltshire, has increasingly involved the RHA and the University Faculty of Medicine as essential partners in its health education programmes as that work has become more specialized. As the scale of the activities has increased from short courses of one or two terms to part-time master's degree courses, so have the RHA and the Faculty of Medicine increased their involvement. This has been important, particularly as a planned feature of all the work at whatever level has been the multiprofessional recruitment of teachers, doctors, health visitors, social workers, health education officers and others, requiring a multidisciplinary input.

Early in 1983 what had been a growing informal working relationship between the University Department of Education and the Wessex RHA was formally recognized in the creation of a new post of Research Fellow in Health Promotion, funded jointly by the Wessex RHA and the Health Education Council. While the Research Fellow was to be based in the University Department of Education, his research and development work would be carried on in both the university and the region.

In a similar way the close cooperation which had developed informally between various departments in the Faculty of Medicine and the Department of Education was recognized and given further impetus by the creation of a new Lectureship in Health Education. Like the Research Fellowship, this was to provide teaching and research support specifically in the area of community health education to complement the existing Education Department strength in school health education. For this reason the post is held jointly in the Departments of Community Medicine and Education, but the person appointed is based in the Department of Education where the major part of the teaching takes place.

These developments have helped to build an infrastructure and create a climate of opinion whereby greater interprofessional cooperation might be achieved at grassroots level. Such cooperation and the implicit role development often involves quite a radical reappraisal of professional norms, relationships and responsibilities. To achieve greater interaction it is essential that the professionals involved recognize the importance of cooperation and take such opportunities as are presented.

A Reorientation of Roles

In the past decade schools as agencies of health education and teachers as practitioners have been enncouraged to look beyond the classroom and to make greater use of and contribute to the communities in which their schools exist. The University of Southampton Department of Education has had a major part in this development as host to successive Schools Health Education Projects.[2] Through these projects teachers have been encouraged to look at the wider aspects of children's health behaviour and to make changes in teaching method and relationships with children in order to extend the relevance of work in the classroom to the community in which the children live. There is good evidence to suggest that these developments have led to considerable change in schools, both in terms of the amount of curriculum time devoted to health education and the variety of methods used by teachers.[3]

Unfortunately such a radical reappraisal of roles, relationships and responsibilities has yet to be paralleled among the health professions, and one of the most important tasks undertaken by the Wessex Positive Health Team in conjunction with the University of Southampton has been to initiate a number of small research projects examining the present and future roles of key health professionals towards the goal of health promotion, and implicit within that aim is the recognition of the importance of interagency cooperation. The roles of a number of key health professionals have been examined, including those of community physicians and health education officers (HEOs), General Practitioners (GPs) and nurses in general practice, and health visitors. A summary of this work follows.

Community Physicians and Health Education Officers

Community physicians and HEOs are the two key health professionals with responsibility for the provision of a coordinated health education service to the community. These two professions above all others in the health services are in a position to foster and support strong interagency cooperation, and for this reason it is essential that they should achieve some measure of consensus in terms of aims, objectives and methods. In addition, because of the coordinating nature of their work, it is essential that both appreciate the wider concepts of health education and fully understand the contribution of the many and various health education agencies — particularly within the education system. Research conducted in Wessex examining the perceptions of health education held by the two groups has indicated that consensus between the two professions may be difficult to achieve.[4]

In the study Health Education Officers believed they had a significant contribution to make to health education in the community as catalysts for activity through a variety of agencies — including those within the education system — but unfortunately many felt hindered by a lack of resources, skills and other support necessary to do so effectively. The community physicians generally interpreted the concept of health education more narrowly than the HEOs, focusing specifically on its application in changing individual lifestyle. This meant, in effect, a concentration of efforts to support individuals and agencies concerned with individual health education rather than support for the work of agencies more concerned with community development and social and environmental change.

Clearly these conflicts of opinion between community physicians and HEOs are likely to have considerable impact on their effectiveness as catalysts for interagency cooperation, and the Wessex study suggests that better understanding and more fruitful cooperation could be achieved through better communication. It is recommended that the two groups engage in more regular structured discussions to facilitate joint approaches to health promotion. This may also encourage the emergence of a consensus view of the health service note in health education. This research has provided an important starting point for change within Wessex and it is anticipated that this will result in better directed and coordinated health education in the community.

The General Practitioner and Practice Nurse

The scope for health education in primary care is becoming increasingly recognized along with the potential for health promotion. However, little information is available at local or national level about how health education is approached in general practice, where success is most likely and what gaps exist. A survey of 200 GPs was conducted in the Wessex Region to identify the level of health education in general practice and to determine the GP's perception of his/her role in relation to the activities and responsibilities of other health care professionals, particularly the practice nurse. The results indicated that the great majority of GPs accepted an important role in health education.[5] Unfortunately, though they accept the role, few GPs appear to make maximum use of the exceptional potential of their regular contact with patients. Most appear reluctant to use their influence to promote health in the absence of disease. Conversely, most have no reservations in offering advice once a diagnosis has been made which can be attributed to illness inducing behaviour. The survey indicates that GPs seem reluctant to make the change from *responding* to established health problems in a preventive way to *anticipating* problems and actively seeking to promote health before problems occur. However, the research highlights a number of developments which may assist this change in that they help to overcome the two main problems of the GP — lack of time and lack of information. These innovations are closely linked to the development of the role of the practice nurse.

Much recent discussion of primary care in the UK has stressed the importance of team work in preventive activities.[6] Most GPs in this survey recognized the importance of interprofessional cooperation in health education, singling out the health visitor as a key figure in primary care, along with the GP. Few, however, recognized a role for the practice nurse.

The practice nurse in the UK is generally regarded as a low-status nursing occupation concerned for example, with the treatment of minor ailments and some immunization procedures. An attractive alternative to this is an extended health promotion role. Given proper training and preparation, a practice nurse could help to organize and run practice-based groups for smoking cessation and weight reduction as well as screening programmes for hypertension, cervical cytology and immunization status. A practice nurse could also help establish a practice information system. This would make information on common risk factors among the practice population more readily available so that the GP could identify 'at-risk' patients, initiate action and follow up progress. Such a structured and coordinated approach to health education through primary care has yet to be seriously attempted on a large scale in the UK, and it is intended that the Wessex study will provide a solid foundation of observations and practical ideas on which such a development may take place.

Health Visitors

Health visitors, like GPs, have great opportunities for health education in their day-to-day contact with clients. Health visitors also have a long tradition as health educators, particularly with respect to young children and parents, and more recently the elderly. Research completed in Wessex indicates that priorities in health visiting are out of step with present health trends.[7] As the pattern of illness in the community as a whole has changed, so too have trends in infant health. Infectious disease and malnourishment were the two most important factors in infant mortality and morbidity twenty-five years ago but these have long been replaced by childhood accidents as the commonest cause of mortality in the 0–5 age group. This study of health visiting practice conducted in the Wessex Region has indicated that present health visiting priorities are still dominated by advice in infant feeding, hygiene and immunization, in that order. Accident prevention rated a poor fourth. The study also highlighted the difficulties associated with health promotion within a problem-oriented service. Client perceptions of the health visitor are like the GPs frequently expressed within a 'problem-solving' perspective and contact time is often used for this purpose. Correspondingly, opportunities for health promotion are reduced. The evidence from the research highlights ways in which health visitors might shift their priorities to match more closely the present perceived needs of the client group. To assist this an innovative model for childhood accident prevention has been developed which it is hoped will provide the basis for a gradual realignment of priorities for this important group of health professionals.

Conclusions

The long-term results of the individual projects cannot yet be assessed but developments at local level in the health service, fostered by this work and the infrastructure and climate of opinion created by developments at regional level offer considerable scope for optimism. In the past two years greater resources than ever before have been made available for health promotion activities. Most DHAs in Wessex now have multidisciplinary groups operating to formulate better planned and more cooperative health promotion activity. Changes of the magnitude experienced in school health education in the past decade now seem set to be paralleled perhaps more widely within the health services in Wessex.

Notes

1 CATFORD, J.C. (1982) *Prospects for Prevention in Wessex* in Wessex Positive Health Team, Winchester, Wessex RHA
2 HEALTH EDUCATION COUNCIL (1983) *Schools Health Education Project 5–13: A Training Manual*, London; HEALTH EDUCATION COUNCIL, SCHOOLS COUNCIL (1980) *HEP 13–18: Co-ordinator's Guide 'Developing Health Education'*, Schools Council, revised version 1983 published by Forbes Publications, London.
3 WILLIAMS, D.T. (1981) *National Survey of Schools in England and Wales*, unpublished survey, University of Southampton.
4 NUTBEAM, D. (1984) 'Health education in the N.H.S.: Differing perceptions of Community Physicians and Health Education Officers', *Health Education Journal*, 43, 4.
5 CATFORD, J.C. and NUTBEAM, D. (1983) 'Prevention in practice: What Wessex General Practitioners are doing', *British Medical Journal*, 288, pp. 832–4.
6 ROYAL COLLEGE OF GENERAL PRACTITIONERS (1984) *Promoting Prevention*, London, RCGP.
7 KAY, E. (1983) *A Model for the Development of Priorities in Health Visiting with Special Respect for the Prevention of Accidents in Childhood*, unpublished M.A. Thesis, University of Southampton.

Some Recent Work at Local Level in Health Education

George Campbell and Peter Farley

At the local level of the smaller local education authorities, along with those sub-divisions of larger LEAs known as 'areas' and the RHA 'districts', there have been changes in recent years, of which the most important has been the devolution of greater powers on to District Health Authorities (DHAs). Unfortunately, such powers are not generally matched in the education system where LEA areas have only limited powers as regards policy and decision-making. While cooperation with their DHA partners is not prevented, the fact that they are of unequal status and power does not facilitate joint operations in health education. Any such intention is complicated by the further fact that boundaries of administrative areas rarely coincide. Nevertheless where there is a will there can also be a way. One Wessex DHA, together with Hampshire Social Services and the Hampshire LEA's Theatre in Education, has successfully funded and run throughout the county a three-year programme of drama presentations in schools on health education themes. This is an example of an interesting and exciting combination of approach and multi-agency local funding. There are other examples in the country but they are not common.

One notable exception to the rule that boundaries rarely coincide is the Isle of Wight LEA whose boundaries coincide exactly with the Isle of Wight DHA. Although the LEA is small, it has all the powers (if not the finance) of a large LEA and so can work with its DHA on equal terms. It is noteworthy how in these circumstances personnel from both the education and health authorities have over the years worked together in the interests of improving the education and health of the Island's people, young and old. Recently, a group representative of this joint interest in health education approached the University of Southampton Department of Education requesting a course in advanced training which would take account of their increasing professional interdependence and need to develop knowledge and skills specific to different work contexts. The resulting health education course being negotiated between the Isle of Wight group and the University is likely to be: based centrally on the Island, part-time for one year, modular in form, the teaching drawing on the accumulated knowledge and expertise of members of various health education project teams based in the Department. Intermodular tasks in curriculum and programme development will be undertaken in the course members' place of work. It will lead to the award of a Postgraduate Certificate, the results being assessed on the basis of the total work assignments. Following this course it is hoped to pilot a revised 5–13 Schools Health Education Project in a selection of the Island's schools, and to monitor the basic health of those children on a regular basis. While at the time of writing these plans have only been discussed in outline, the fact that the three main partners, the Isle of Wight LEA, the DHA and the University of Southampton, can work together productively towards agreed objectives in health education and health promotion is itself a significant achievement.

At the very localized level of the school and its neighbourhood the health education scene in England and Wales is characterized by local initiatives which differ not only from one LEA area to another but also from school to school. In this country it is possible to have two schools geographically close to each other, externally similar in every respect, and yet within having quite different curricula and methods of working. One school may be consciously teaching health education regularly to all its pupils through a variety of subjects, the work of the teachers supplemented by contributions from outside agencies. The other school may have as a deliberate policy a curriculum which excludes the teaching of health education for all pupils.

The greatest contribution to the local growth and development of health education in schools in England and Wales, Scotland and Northern Ireland has been without doubt the pioneer work of the Schools Health Education Project (SHEP) 5–13 and more recently 13–18. The extent of the success of SHEP 13–18 can be gauged by the realization that no fewer than fifty out of 109 LEAs in England and Wales have involved their schools in the project since its inception in 1980. In Scotland, which has worked closely with England and Wales, almost all the regions are now involved; and in Northern Ireland, all the Education and Library Boards.

There is no doubt that the strategies and methods of working which emerged from the trials phase have proved successful. In particular was the recognition of the individuality of schools and the need to provide an approach sufficiently flexible to fit in with the school rather than something to be superimposed. To support this approach there was the recognition also that a health education coordinator should be identified in each school and then trained for the task initially through a series of workshops designed by the SHEP team for that purpose. Finally, in recognition of the power vested in the headteacher which could be used for or against health education in school, headteachers' seminars were established. In these, the heads were confronted with key questions designed to tax their understanding of the project, their degree of commitment to it and the practical implications for their staff and pupils if their schools took part. For those schools who decided in favour, a *Coordinator's Guide* was provided to assist at every step in the development of the work in the school, and to provide a basic agenda for each of the workshops conducted by the SHEP team.[1] The *Coordinator's Guide* is also designed to be used by the coordinator back in school with colleagues. The autonomy and individuality of schools respected in the approach of the project as a whole is reflected in the different patterns of use of the *Guide* by coordinators in school. Coordinators are encouraged to make their own judgments with regard to the extent to which they select from the guide (adaptation) or use it in full as originally conceived (adherence). The contents suggest practical tasks as well as provide structured means to address important issues such as aims methods and priorities. With the school/community interface particularly in mind, there are suggestions and tools offered which seek community views of pupils' needs and encourage opportunities for community involvement in health education activities both on and off the school site. At its best, the use of the *Guide* by coordinators with their colleagues not only enhances the coordination of health education but meshes closely curriculum development with the personal and professional development of the staff involved in a school-based setting. Over the period 1980–83, which marked the Dissemination Phase, three-stage workshops have been conducted in most parts of the UK.

In April 1983, having almost concluded the Dissemination Phase, the SHEP 13–18 team held a conference for trainers to review progress and collectively distil ideas on how future training initiatives could best be supported. The conference report sets out the detail culled from the experience of those with whom the team had worked in various parts of the country.[2]

Predictably, the critical factors which emerged were those which have already been discussed in respect of other innovative work in health education. Considering them in order from national to local level, they were as follows:

1 *The attitude of government and whether policies exist which promote health education*
   This is true at all levels. Clearly if a national policy exists which is backed by finance and other supportive measures, the process of developing health education programmes in school and community throughout the country becomes that much easier, and more likely to bear fruit. Similarly, if at regional and LEA levels supportive policies exist, even if there is no overarching national policy, health education in school and community may still prosper. If no supportive policies exist at any level, the task of promoting health education is then much more difficult, depending as it does on 'pioneers', enthusiasts and pressure groups who may be able to

influence local or regional authorities into rethinking attitudes and policies.

2 *The support of national organizations*

The support of the Schools Council and the Health Education Council through their policies and resources has been crucial to the achievement of progress to date. At an operational level the active support of TACADE personnel and the recognition of the inter-dependence of much of their work has been a source of strength. It is also apparent that much implicit support comes through the work of other colleagues in the field of personal and social education working on parallel if not converging courses. Examples are Active Tutorial Work and Lifeskills Teaching Programmes.[3]

3 *The dependence upon support at local level*

(i) It is important that the school's curricular policy recognizes health education as an important component. The attitude of the headteacher is still crucial. Is the headteacher supportive or neutral (which may be interpreted as latent hostility)? How clearly and efficiently the school is organized internally is important, as is the quality of the health education team. Good internal communications are essential. The coordinator is the key person. His/her status in the school and personal qualities that can be brought to bear on the task will contribute much to the progress of health education there.

(ii) The school-community link is important. The major considerations are:

The strength, representation and organization of local networks, and willingness and ability to support school health education.

The need for clarification of roles in community health education as well as in school health education so as to know 'who does what? where? when? and how?' The need for training courses (in addition to SHEP workshops); short courses for individual professional groups seem to be preferred in early stages, with multiprofessional recruitment at later or more advanced stages. The lack of group work skills is still a serious impediment to effective cooperation.

The recognition of the education advisory officer (the adviser) as a key link between school and LEA no less important than that of the health education officer with the DHA. Furthermore, in such innovatory schemes as SHEP workshops it is essential that the adviser be present on all occasions, to support and legitimize the work of the teachers.

Teacher centres and health education centres provide complementary services for school teams enabling coordinators and others to meet and exchange ideas, thrash out problems and provide mutual support. Again, the adviser and HEO are potential catalysts in the development of future work, both at the centre and through following up at the schools.

Headteachers and school governors must be kept up-to-date officially about developments in health education, especially examples of good practice in health education, county guidelines in health education, etc.

Parents as a key community partner must also be kept up-to-date with developments and wherever possible involved actively in the process of their child's health education.

Overall, however, is the need for school policy with regard to health education to be viewed in relation to LEA and DHA policy; it cannot work successfully for long in isolation.

Notes

1 SCHOOLS COUNCIL (1980) *HEP 13–18: Coordinator's Guide 'Developing Health Education'*, Schools Council, revised version 1984 published by Forbes Publications, London.
2 CHARLES WISE (Ed.) (1983) *Health Education Project 13–18 Report*, Health Education Unit, University of Southampton.
3 'Active Tutorial Work' is published in six volumes by Basil Blackwell in association with Lancashire County Council; 'Lifeskills' Teaching Programmes by B. HOPSON and M. SEALLY are published in two packs by Lifeskills Associates, Leeds.

Appendix

The International Seminar on School Health Education

(i) Background

This volume is the result of an international seminar which took place in Southampton in 1981 and of subsequent work (up to 1983) which has been reported back by the participants from their respective countries.

A number of events and developments combined to indicate the *school-community interface* as a problem area in school health education requiring early attention. The WHO Conference at Gent in September 1980 concluded with three specific recommendations, all of which identified acute school-community concerns:

1 Consideration should be given to the development of a theoretical model which would serve to illustrate the dynamic relationship between different elements and components in society which interact to determine the quality nature and persistence of constraints affecting education for health.
2 All necessary measures should be taken to create openness and dialogue between schools and their communities.
3 Investment should be concentrated on integrating the principles of health education into the preparation and training of all professional groups involved with community work.

The Schools Council Health Education Projects, which had recently moved to Southampton University, were already anticipating the next series of strategies to follow their three-stage workshops, and independently identified effective school-community coordinated health education programmes as a priority.

Finally, for some time, in-service policies in the Southampton region involving teachers and community field-workers had been highlighting the need both to harness important community resources (knowledge and expertise) in the planning and/or teaching of health education programmes and to understand more clearly the problems preventing more effective cooperation.

Discussions with colleagues during visits to several Western European countries and subsequent correspondence with other colleagues in other parts of Europe and in North America confirmed a strong interest in the school-community interface as that area of concern with school health education which they would wish to pursue together.

The nuclear planning team at Southampton University — George Campbell, Peter Kelly and Trefor Williams — then set to work to plan a seminar with the following features:

1   linking in with current work and attempting to follow on from the 1980 WHO Gent Conference;
2   a focus on issues in Europe and North America because of common elements in their respective cultures and associated problems;
3   a maximum of forty participants to work in small groups concentrating on the discussion of important issues. This would underline the importance of everyone's contribution, and assist the emergence of significant national differences of emphasis, rather than bland general statements of goodwill;
4   invitations to attend and prepare papers to two leading health educators in each of the countries of Western Europe and North America. It was envisaged that the numbers would be made up by six representatives from the host country to assist in the organization and running of the seminar;
5   papers raising key issues would be circulated to participants before the seminar, which in turn would require only short 'clarifying sessions' before the issues were taken up by the working groups;
6   a short statement on the present situation of school health education in each of their countries, and the particular topics they would wish to study at the seminar, to be provided by the participants.

The response to the outline plan was very favourable from national and international bodies, and some funding was promised by the British Council.

The seminar took as its starting point that familiar boundary which marks the differences between school health education on the one hand, and home or neighbourhood health education on the other; between teacher perceptions, parent perceptions and the perceptions of community workers in the health, social and medical fields of what school health education is and what it should be. Four aspects were selected for detailed consideration:

1   constraints on school-community interaction;
2   policies, strategies and methodologies;
3   professional training — initial and in-service;
4   community involvement — professional and lay;

In this way it was hoped the seminar would move towards a clearer definition of *models of school-community interaction in the field of school health education* as a means of understanding and overcoming the present constraints.

Thirty-eight health educators attended from sixteen countries including the UK. The various disciplinary backgrounds included medical, nursing and administrative, as well as educational, and reflected experience not only at national level but at regional and local levels too. Since the working groups were already planned with an international representation, the variety of disciplinary backgrounds and levels of experience promised to provide valuable additional perspectives. The four working groups under their leaders Donald Iverson (USA), Jos v. Hameron (Netherlands), Heather Hyde (UK), Eugene Donoghue (Ireland) were fed key issues and questions from the papers which were further refined in the short plenary sessions which preceded group discussions. The four rapporteurs who recorded discussion and produced reports were: Mary Holmes, Peter Farley, Lewis Slack and Charles Wise (all of UK).

(ii) Working Group Discussions

Part 1. Understanding the Constraints on School-Community Interaction: Discussion

Experience of the relationships between school and community varied enormously. However, after considerable discussion a number of common features emerged:

1 It is essential to define 'community' in unambiguous and meaningful terms with respect to 'level' i.e., is it 'the community in general' which could mean at national level or at the other extreme the very local community which sends its children to a particular school? Community needs to be defined in operational terms before meaningful relationships can be discussed.

2 Associated with the problem of the definition of community is the problem of boundaries. There are the boundaries imposed by schools or the community around their perimeter; their strength or weakness depending on school or community perceptions of respective roles: teacher, parent, community health, medical and social service personnel, members of the public. Strong boundaries reflecting strong role definition discourage cooperation; schools, in such circumstances, experience little outside influence. Weak boundaries, on the other hand, allow much more two-way traffic and scope for cooperation. Complicating the picture are the more subtle and less observable boundaries around different cultural and

sub-cultural groups, e.g., religious, ethnic, peer groups, etc. which reflect their different values and attitudes, in particular towards health and health education. For instance, the development in children of knowledge, responsibility and competency with regard to their own health may increase tension and conflict with parents, where the latter believe that family life and values are threatened. Similarly, health may be a difficult concept for teenagers to entertain when health education, in its attempts to project a realistic picture, concentrates on 'problems' and a problem-centred approach at a stage when the teenager is more concerned with 'a positive self-image'.

3 The incidence of successful health education programmes is higher in primary schools than in secondary, perhaps as a result of the greater degree of permeability of school-community boundaries at primary school level.

4 The practical difficulties of involving 'clients' in the identification of their needs and priorities, which, ideally, should form the starting point of policy and programme planning. Difficulties become accentuated when working with children and socially disadvantaged groups who have little experience or tradition of taking initiatives. There is, moreover, the danger of emphasizing the individual's interests at the expense of the group or community; hence the overriding need to maintain a balanced and flexible perspective.

5 Even if school and community agencies achieve a consensus on joint policies, the resources (human and financial) may not be available to implement those policies. Additionally, if this is a local initiative, political pressures at regional or national levels may further inhibit progress. In the absence of this support, it is doubtful if the collaborative effort could be usefully sustained.

6 In the promotion of 'models of good practice' at local level, national policies need to supplement national funding with a local financial contribution as an aid to motivation. A financial stake encourages active involvement!

7 The danger that financial and political pressures to produce results may distort or change those parts of the health education process considered to be valuable but not very amenable to measurement, e.g., self-esteem, personal competency, individual autonomy.

8 The legitimacy of the experimental approach in health education is a problem, especially where issues of health are confused with issues of social control. It becomes an acute source of concern when faced with such emotive matters as smoking or solvent misuse among schoolchildren.

9 In spite of reaching agreement on what constitutes some of the main health education issues between school and community, it is

important to continue the study of *the presentation of health education across the school-community boundary as a complex problem requiring clearer resolution.*

Part 2. Policies, Strategies and Methods of Achieving Understanding and Cooperation: Discussion

1   The PRECEDE model quoted by Kolbe (see Figure 1) provides a valuable insight into the context of school health education, and the factors which must influence policies, strategies and methods across boundaries. The consideration of such factors could enable the various agencies involved to identify and clarify their roles in the process of formulating collaborative policies. The model has the further advantage of identifying important items for discussion, but can leave implementation to local level initiatives without the need for dependence on a national strategy. It also assists the conceptualization of health education as being different activities in different contexts but with a constant concern for the underlying educative process.

2   Who should initiate a policy of school-community cooperation? Schools as agents of the community should perhaps be the prime movers at local level in encouraging and facilitating a more participatory partnership. An imponderable, however, is the 'terms of reference' of schools and other community agencies, and whether their policies permit them to participate in joint planning and to reconsider their roles in health education. It is essential that the educational view of 'what school health education is or ought to be' should be debated in the light of other community views such as those of the health, medical and social services (statutory and voluntary) as well as religious and political interests.

3   The appropriate means of accountability for cross-boundary, multiagency and mixed interest group activities must be ensured. At present, different groups are accountable, if at all, in different ways.

4   There is a need to shift away from the traditional agent-client relationship to a more 'equal partnership' with the client, in order to clarify viable joint policies and appropriate action. In the light of the prevalent danger of basing policies on perceptions of the problem other than the client's, there is a need for more 'client-centred' health education. In line with this there is clearly a need for the re-education of some policy-makers and field-workers. The parents' role is a particular issue to be resolved, not only in the specific school health education context but in a wider sense, as some governments involve parents more actively in school govern-

Figure 1. The PRECEDE Model

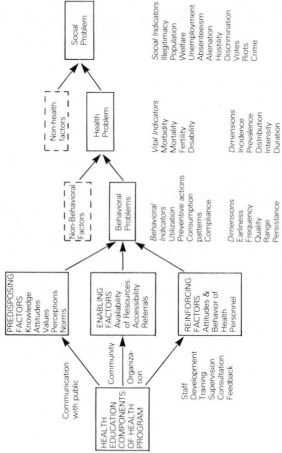

Approximate relationships among 'objects of interests' in the planning and evaluation of health education.

Source: Green, L.S. (1974) 'Toward cost-benefit evaluations of health education: Some concepts, methods, and examples', *Health Education Monographs*, Vol. 2, Supplement 1, pp. 34–64.

ment and in the overview of the curriculum. This could work for or against health education.

5 In times of financial cut-back and limited resources, priorities should be established, of which one might be identifying 'at-risk' groups and what their special needs are, rather than the population as a whole. One possible strategy might be a training in decision-making skills for disadvantaged groups who are unable to implement 'healthy' decisions.

6 A suggested common policy ground among different countries might be a focus on 'health related behaviours' which could then be pursued together by schools and their communities, the latter comprising the various agencies as well as the community in the broader sense. Such a focus would enable roles and tasks to be identified in association with the clarification of a local epidemiology and priority of needs. An important task would be the resolution of different perceptions of needs and priorities by the various interest groups: pupils, parents, teachers, doctors, etc.

7 There is a need for 'broad spectrum' planning, in the UK, for example, by community physicians in their district community health councils particularly in the light of 1982 NHS reorganization. The purpose and nature of contributions to joint activities need to be identified at an early stage, rather than recruited on an ad hoc basis as crises arise.

8 The USA National Health Programme, 'The Objectives for the Nation', provides a good illustration of the interlocking of national and local policies in health education. National policy with regard to the funding of health education programmes is based on the epidemiological evidence. Each of the states is provided with a person whose task is to identify and support proposed health programmes, all of which must be concerned with one or more of the identified objectives. Such large-scale funding is seen as one way of influencing national 'lifestyle', and since this applies especially to young people, the school health education programmes are seen as important. At local level community involvement is ensured by encouraging voluntary organizations to 'invest' financially. In addition, local communities are free to operate health education programmes in their own way, provided they meet the identified objectives.

9 The more prevalent European pattern is for different stages of policy development to be found in different countries. If the stages are broadly distinguished as 'preventive', 'positive pioneer intervention' and 'the development of systems', these may all be encountered in varying degrees of development, often superimposed on each other. For instance, some countries use 'disease warnings' or promote behaviour change by instilling fear through

advertisements or 'educational films' in spite of increasing evidence that such effects are not long lasting. Most countries still use 'positive pioneers' drawn from voluntary and statutory agencies to inspire and initiate curriculum development. Some countries now have school health education plans drawn up at either national or local levels, in varying degrees of sophistication or elaboration, for schools to use if they so wish.

10   On the ethical question of the legitimacy of experimental methods in health education there is a consensus view that while experimentation should not be encouraged, the reality of it and its possible contribution to important generalizable health knowledge should be accepted, with the proviso that it might not be the most appropriate focus for health educators and researchers.

11   There is a need to 'sell' health education where perceptions may be negative and health education is seen as disruptive or subversive. This is particularly so when such views are held by high-status, influential individuals.

12   In some countries there is a renewed emphasis on science, mathematics and technology in the curriculum. Does this argue for a closer alliance between health education and physical science, perhaps integrated in 'health science'; and a corresponding distancing from the 'affective' domain and such areas of study as life-skills? In times of social and industrial change and unemployment how is the right balance established between the affective curriculum and the science curriculum, both of which are needed to regenerate complementary facets of society: the personal and social and the economic?

13   There is need for the systematic identification, diffusion and dissemination of good practices by national agencies in particular, in order to inform developments at provincial or regional and local levels.

14   Methods of promoting effective school and community interaction include:

   (i)   interprofessional in-service training — often suggested but not as often carried out;

   (ii) local liaison groups;

  (iii) a health convention or a project, involving the community: other professionals, voluntary 'pioneers' and parents;

  (iv) health fairs organized by the students themselves;

   (v) school involvement with the handicapped and/or young children;

  (vi) 'need assessment tools', i.e., questionnaires to pupils, teachers and parents on what they think are important health issues:

(vii)   parent-teacher association talks by a doctor or community health educator;
(viii) local media, e.g., radio programme series and campaigns at popular listening times;
(ix)   police can sometimes be used, with care, on certain issues in some countries. This depends to some extent on the image of the police in the community and the age of the pupils;
(x)   projects in which pupils visit local agencies. Care needs to be taken that the agencies are not overburdened with visits.

Part 3 Professional Training: Discussion

There was considerable variation in the extent to which health education was included in teacher training. While in-service training was considered most important, the initial training period provided an early opportunity for student teachers to be sensitized to the need for continuing the process. As yet few countries seem to recognize this in their initial or in-service provision.

1   The serious 'falling rolls' situation which is likely to persist for some years in Western European countries will place a greater emphasis on in-service as opposed to initial training since there will be fewer openings for newly qualified teachers. It may also cause teachers to look beyond the subject specialisms in which they were originally trained in order to make more flexible and varied subject offerings. This may further encourage them to examine other facets of their role, and new skills, in particular those concerned with social relationships.

2   Teachers may find difficulty in participating in experiential work. For instance, they may be prepared to discuss group work, but, for a variety of reasons, be unwilling or unable to participate in it. In-service training programmes must be sensitive to such difficulties and assist teachers to overcome them, if school-based training and curriculum development are to succeed.

3   There are political implications in the advocacy of certain strategies and methods, such as 'self-empowerment', which may be interpreted as running counter to social aspirations and the national interest. Self-empowerment also needs to be squared with possible expectations of health education programmes to produce behaviour change.

4   The status and origin of training demand careful scrutiny. Training may be coordinated at national, provincial or local level to

ensure compatibility with existing teacher or other professional training policies. The health educator may need to question or criticize, and adopt a role which may be incompatible with existing or traditional training systems. There is, therefore, an important role for an independent body, such as a university, in building adaptable school-community training bridges. Where the latter are linked to award-bearing courses, these shoud be viewed in wider terms than purely academic, and their examinations not only in terms of what can be measured.

5 Opportunities should be provided in initial training courses for student teachers and trainee professionals to develop their own autonomy. The retrained mid-career and experienced teacher and other professionals could be a major resource in assisting in the renegotiation and reshaping of school-community health education programmes. With enlightened retraining together, their influence upon each other could enhance individual self-esteem and self-empowerment, extending it to their respective professional groups.

6 A focal theme for retraining should, perhaps, be 'education for life-skills'. Several factors which could facilitate its acceptance are:
  (i)   initial and in-service training which supports, extends and applies the concept of life-skills education;
  (ii)   the extent to which new entrants to the profession and experienced teachers in post see themselves as change-agents and innovators;
  (iii) an emphasis on defining life-skills education in terms of both problem-solving and improving capabilities in order that it is seen to be an integral part of mainstream education;
  (iv)   official support and encouragement by policy-makers and teachers' professional organizations.

7 The following approaches should enable some lowering of the threat-threshold to teachers in inviting other health professionals to participate in school health education who may see the educative process differently:
  (i)   schools should emphasize that they share a mutual concern for the health of young people and that they are not competing but looking for common ground of mutual support within which to articulate this concern;
  (ii)   there should be public recognition of the substantial contribution to school health education made by teachers and community agencies, each offering a unique and expert contribution. Each group or individual should be assured of the essential complementary nature of their contribution.

8   Health professionals may also act as advisers rather than as teachers. They provide a different, yet valid perspective.

9   The context in which the health professional operates is crucial to how she/he sees health education, e.g., the nurse in the hospital (clinical role), in the clinic (counselling role) and in the school (preventive role). We must be aware of these different perspectives, how the roles differ and the significance of the differences.

10 Suggested early stages in deciding on interservice or interagency training plans:

   (i)   evaluate what has been done and not done and what the further needs are;

   (ii) identify and evaluate existing practice and what can be learned from it.

(Such evaluation can be done formally or informally, using, for example, the 'health education underground'. But the health educator has a clear function in such an evaluation and can take the lead.)

   (iii) identify training needs (more realistic in a cooperative framework than in an independent, isolated one).

Part 4. Discussion The Special Role of the School Health Service:

The Present Position   It is not possible to give more than an impression of the main features of the school health service in a number of the countries represented.

In the UK the position of the health service in schools is very variable, but quite often the school nurse knows the children well and plays some part in health education programmes. 'Pastoral Committees' of school staff, health visitors and education welfare officers, where they exist, perform a useful function in monitoring children's personal development.

In Belgium the school health service has two methods of providing health education: (1) by giving talks and individual medical counselling; (2) by identifying and planning programmes. In addition, and independently of the school health service, some schools are working with new health education curriculum materials. In a health convention recently promoted by a doctor, young people and adults met together to discuss each other's views. No doctors, however, were involved in the actual convention!

The USA uses school nurses in the health service and retrains them as nurse practitioners. For individual children, follow-up for treatment is often only taken where handicaps or defects affect the child's learning.

School health service personnel and teachers need to know each other. There are communication problems within the health service reflecting the hierarchy among doctors and nurses and the relationship of both to teachers and parents. There is, too, the problem of professional confidentiality.

Future Possibilities More effective cooperation between the school health service and the schools might be promoted by:-

1   involving the school nurse rather than the doctor in routine screening procedures;
2   using doctors rather than nurses to persuade the headteacher to introduce programmes of health education into the schools;
3   persuading parents to take a more informed interest in school medical examinations;
4   school nurses and doctors being available for discussion with pupils (at mutually agreed times) on whether or not to seek further advice, and parents being involved in examinations;
5   There is a need to preserve and respect confidentiality as more parties gain access to more information;
6   Nurses and doctors should be *consultants* to health education work but not necessarily determine it. Similarly health educators should be *consulted* by doctors and nurses. For both groups there is a need for 'referents' to ensure consistency of message and this would include reference to trainers;
7   There is need for evaluation, assessment, clarification and accountability for medical interventions;
8   The issue of cooperation with the school health service is made more pressing by developments in several countries which seek the integration of the handicapped or those with other chronic conditions into the 'normal' school.

In Norway many younger doctors would like to be involved in health education for children, and would prefer to leave the screening to the nurses. Instead of duplicating the national health service with a school health service, schools should teach more about the effective use of the national health service. The school health service should develop a declared policy in relation to schools, and school nurses should have adequate training which should include a school placement and some understanding of the curriculum. Two related key questions are:

1   Given the medical dominance and sporadic contact which often seems to characterize the school health service, how can the service effectively cooperate with other agencies?
2   What kind of structure does the school health service need in order to best fulfil its four-fold support function, viz:
    (i)   information giving;
    (ii) integration of health education into screening programmes;
    (iii) transmission of specific skills, i.e., in first aid;
    (iv) concern with medical aspects of the learning situation.

The study of information on the organization and operation of the school health system in a number of countries — Luxembourg, Denmark, Finland, USA, Switzerland and UK — revealed three common factors:

1　Organization: if the school health service is really integrated into the school system, then it effectively supports health education initiatives;
2　Role expectations: there is a possibility that health professionals adopt a problem/pathology-focused approach, and that they perceive health education as synonymous with health promotion which, manifestly, it is not;
3　Communication: health professionals may need post-qualification training in ways of working effectively with young people.

(iii)　Overview

Stanley Mitchell

A number of important points were identified for further consideration, and as possible directions for future work, some of which are taken up in Parts 4 and 5 of this volume:

1　Under 'representation', there was some imbalance in that the school health and medical services were more strongly represented from the Continent than from the UK or USA, while educationists were more strongly represented from the UK and USA, Administrators, members of government (national or local), 'lively journalists' and reactionaries were unrepresented.
2　Although the working groups conducted detailed discussion of all the main issues and resolved many of them, there was, nevertheless, some advantage in reaffirming the importance of the following:
　　the parents' role in health education;
　　the client's role in health education;
　　the scientific aspects of health education;
　　the need for the school health service to be 'educated about education';
　　the need for effective coordination at national or regional levels to offset the sometimes competing claims of piecemeal developments at local level;
　　the need to successfully market the concept of health education.
3　There was some danger that the following might be underestimated:
　　the justifiable insecurity of other professionals with whom cooperation is envisaged, particularly in times of social change and economic cut-back;

the creation of an 'in-language' in health education which may not be comprehensible to those it is intended to help — 'meanings and messages must be clear'.

4 The wisdom of the Schools Council Health Education Project philosophy is not questioned. Is this a healthy state?

5 'Results in improved health are ultimately what we are after.'

(iv) Membership (Additional to Contributors)

DENMARK Dr Majken Kristensen, School Doctor, Municipality of Copenhagen, Hestveg 2, 2900 Charlottenlund.
Chirstin Plate, County Health Visitor, County of Copenhagen, Social Welfare Centre of the County Council, Huidoureveg 438, 2650 Huidore.

FRANCE Mme Francoise Buhl, Delegue General, Comité Francais d'Education pour La Santé, 9 rue Newton, 75116 Paris.

GREECE Dr Pavlos Ghikas, School Medical Officer (Child-Psychiatrist), Ministry of Social Services, 19 Aristotelous Str., Athens.

IRELAND Mr John Condon, Education Officer, Health Education Bureau, 7 Ely Place, Dublin 2.
Mr Eugene Donoghue, Education and Training Officer, Health Education Bureau, 7 Ely Place, Dublin 2.

LUXEMBOURG Dr Margot Muller, Médecin Chef de Service, Direction de la Santé, Service de Médecine Scolaire, 37 rue Glesener, Luxembourg.

NETHERLANDS Dr Jos van Hameren, Director of the Dutch Service Centre for Health Education, John F. Kennedylaan 101, 3981 GB Bunnik.
Dr Olga M. Teunissen, Advisory Committee for Curriculum Development H.E., Prinses Irenestraat 6, 6611 BH Overasselt.

NORWAY Mr Ole S. Myrnes, Assistant Secretary, Department of Church and Education, Box 8119 Dep., Oslo 1.

SWITZERLAND Dr Karin Butschi, Doctor in Medicine, Youth's Health Service, Service de Santé de la Jeunesse, 11 Glacis-de-Rive, 1207 Geneva.
Ms Ariane Randell, Public Health Nurse, Service Santé de la Jeunesse, Case postale 374, 1211 Geneve 3.

UNITED KINGDOM Mr John Brierley, HMI with national responsibility for health education, DES, 11 Park Place, Bristol.
Mrs Heather Hyde, Education Officer, Health Education Council.

WEST GERMANY Herr Manfred Lehmann, Dipl, Soz., ORR, Bundeszentrale fur Gesundheitliche Aufklarung, Postfach 91 0152.

LOCAL Southampton and South West Hampshire Health Education Service: Mrs Pat Christmas, District Health Education Officer; Dr Stephen MacKeith, Health Education Consultant.

UNIVERSITY OF SOUTHAMPTON Professor Peter Kelly, Dean of the Faculty of Educational Studies; Mr Lewis Slack and Mr Charles Wise, Research Fellows, Health Education Unit, Department of Education.

(v)   School Health Education in the Countries Represented

Before the Seminar returns were received on a short questionnaire previously circulated which was intended to provide information on:

1   the state of school health education in each of the countries represented under a number of key headings, e.g., level of provision, teacher training, legislation, etc.;
2   the important issues facing school health education in each country;
3   those issues which could be most usefully pursued at the Seminar.

The information to which all participants had access during the Seminar is set out in Table 1. (The representative of Portugal was unable to attend.)

Appendix

Table 1   School Health Education in the Countries Represented (1981)

Questions	Belgium	Denmark	Finland	France	Ireland	Luxembourg
1. Is there curriculum development in the field?						
1.1 nationally?	Yes. Under discussion.	Yes	Yes	Yes	Yes	Yes. Primary and pre-school.
1.2 regionally?	—	No	No	Yes	Yes	—
1.3 locally?	—	Yes	No	Yes	Yes	—
2. Is it directed at						
2.1 junior school?	Yes	Yes	Yes	Yes	Yes	Yes
2.2 secondary school?	No	Yes	Yes	Yes	Yes	Yes (some)
3. Is its product						
3.1 teacher guides?	Yes	Yes	Yes	Yes	Yes	Yes
3.2 pupil materials?	Yes	Yes	Yes	Yes	Yes (limited)	Yes
4.1 Is community involvement or support a feature?	No (under consideration)	Yes	Some: varies locally	Yes	Yes	No
4.2 If so, how is it defined?	—	By local parent boards' approval of the curriculum and pupil materials.	—	No general pattern. Depends upon local goodwill.	To promote contact with school. To advise on health education programme.	—
5.1 In-service modules for teachers?	Yes being planned.	No	Occasional	No	Yes	Occasional
5.2 Recruitment from other professional groups?	—	—	Yes	Yes	Yes	Occasional
6. Initial teacher training include health education?	No	Yes	Yes	No	No	Yes (option)
6.1 for all students?	—	Yes	No	—	—	—
6.2 for those intending to specialize?	—	—	Yes	—	—	—
7.1 Legal framework for teaching health education in school?	No	Yes	No	No	No	No
7.2 Implicit in education policies?	No	—	Yes	No	No	—
8. Important issues in development of health education?	—	1 Dental care 2 Food and eating habits 3 Smoking 4 Alcohol 5 Sex 6 Hygiene	1 No time in curriculum for health education. 2 Strengthening health education objectives in school. 3 Developing external cooperation.	1 National policy. 2 Teacher training. 3 Training of health educators. 4 Community coordination.	1 School organization. 2 Teacher training. 3 Material development. 4 Pre-service training.	1 School/community interaction. 2 Increasing teacher awareness.
9. Issues most useful to pursue in the Seminar?		Excesses of above. Learning to live in a changing society.	As above	Evaluation	Teacher training	1 Defining role of school health service. 2 Promotion of school-community interaction.

Note: — Indicates no reply or not applicable.

School Health Education in the Countries Represented (1981)

Netherlands	Norway	Portugal	Scotland	Spain	Switzerland	USA	United Kingdom
Yes	Yes	Yes	Yes	Yes	No	Yes	Yes
Yes	No	—	Yes	—	Yes	Yes	Yes (some)
Yes	No	—	Yes	—	Yes	Yes	Yes (some)
Yes	Yes	Yes	Yes	Yes	Yes	Yes	Yes
Yes	Yes	Yes	Yes	No	Yes	Yes	Yes
Yes	Yes	No	Yes	Yes	No	Yes	Yes
Yes	Yes	Yes (few)	Little	Yes	Yes	Yes	Yes
Yes	No	—	No	No	Yes	Yes	Partly
Health organizations provide financial support and materials.	—	—	—	—	Various representative committees	Individuals and groups assist in planning and implementation. Coordinated agencies.	Left to local initiative; therefore 'patchy'.
Yes	No	No	Yes	No	No	Yes	Yes
Partly	—	—	Little	—	—	Yes	Yes
Yes	Yes (little)	Yes (primary)	Yes	No	Very little	Yes (elected)	Little
No	Yes	Yes	Yes	—	Yes	—	—
Yes	Yes	—	—	—	—	Yes	—
Yes	Yes	No	No	Yes	No	Yes in some States.	No
—	Yes	No	Yes	Yes	No	—	Yes
1 Legislation about comprehensive school health education. 2 Curriculum development. 3 Innovative teacher training.		1 National policy. 2 Curriculum development (primary). 3 Coordinating school and community. 4 Increase community involvement.	1 Health education for all pupils. 2 Teachers' lack of confidence. 3 LEAs' lack of commitment.	1 Health education as preparation for life. 2 Community-school interaction.	1 Role of school health service in health education. 2 Lack of qualified personnel and of material resources. 3 Poor coordination and cooperation between professional groups.	1 Clarifying perceptions of health education. 2 Improving skills of interchange. 3 Coordinating schools and community at a national level.	1 Clarifying health education as an important priority. 2 Defining success in health education. 3 Clarifying health education professionals' contribution.
1 Implementation strategies in schools. 2 Teacher training.		1 In-service training for teachers and health professionals. 2 Community involvement. 3 Strategies of implementation.	1 Building up teacher confidence.	1 School-community interaction.	1 Coordination and cooperation among professional services.	As 8 above.	As 8 above.

Notes on Contributors

George Campbell is Coordinator of Advanced Courses in Health Education in the Department of Education, University of Southampton, England.

Professor Martin V. Covington is Professor of Psychology at the Lawrence Hall of Science, University of California at Berkeley, USA.

Peter Farley is Director of the Schools Health Education Projects 13–18 and 16–19, based in the Health Education Unit, Department of Education, University of Southampton, England.

Arne Hauknes is Head of Secretariat, National Council on Smoking and Health, Oslo, Norway.

Mary Holmes is the former Senior Inspector of Schools with national responsibility for health education in England and Wales. Currently she is Visiting Fellow in the Department of Education, University of Southampton, England.

Dr Donald C. Iverson is Special Assistant to the Director, US Office of Health Information and Health Promotion, Washington D.C., USA.

Dr Lloyd J. Kolbe is the former Director of Evaluation, National Centre for Health Education, School Health Education Project, San Bruno, California. Currently he is Director of Health Information, US Office of Health Information, Department of Health and Human Services, Washington D.C., USA.

Lea Maes is Scientific Assistant (Sociology), Department of Social Medicine, University of Gent, Belgium.

Dr Colette Menard is a psychologist in the Department of Studies and Research, National Health Education Committee, Paris, France.

Stanley C. Mitchell is Director of the Scottish Health Education Group, Edinburgh, Scotland.

Dr Pilar Najera is Head of the Health Education Section, Ministry of Health and Social Security, Madrid, Spain.

Donald Nutbeam is Research Fellow in Health Promotion, Department of Education, University of Southampton, England.

Donald Reid is Assistant Director (Schools), Health Education Council, London, England.

Dr Matti Rimpela is Associate Professor in Medical Sociology, Department of Public Health Science, University of Helsinki, Finland.

Dr Hans Saan is Coordinator of Training in Health Education, Hogere School voor Gezondheidszorg, Utrecht, Netherlands.

Dr Herbert D. Thier is Associate Director, Lawrence Hall of Science, University of California at Berkeley, USA.

Dr Keith Tones is Principal Lecturer in Health Education, School of Hospitality and Home Economics, Leeds Polytechnic, and a Council Member of the Health Education Council, London, England.

Trefor Williams is Director of the Health Education Research and Development Unit, Department of Education, University of Southampton, England.

Index

Aar, L.E. *et al.*, 124n4 and n5
academic aspects
  of school life, 11
Act Relating to the Basic School (1969,
  Norway), 118–19
Act Relating to Schools (1860, Norway),
  117–18
Active Tutorial Work (ATW) project,
  186–7, 189, 206, 207n3
agricultural extension service
  and health education in Spain, 148–9
Ahlstrom, S., 101, 105
Ahlstrom, S. *et al.*, 101, 105
alcohol, 9, 101–2, 105, 194
allergic disorders
  in Finland, 100
Alliance Nationale des Mutualités
  Chrétiennes, 90
American Academy of Pediatrics, 33,
  41n21
American Alliance for Health, Physical
  Education, and Recreation, 33, 41n18
American Association for Health, Physical
  Education, and Recreation, 37, 42n41
American Association of School
  Administrators, 31
American Medical Association (AMA), 33,
  41n13–16, 43n53, n54 and n56
American Public Health Association, 33,
  41n20
American School Health Association, 33,
  41n19
American School Health Education Study,
  11
Anderson, C.L. and Creswell, W.H.,
  41n24

Asian Patients, 127, 129, 130
Aston, University of, 193–4
ATW
  see Active Tutorial Work project

Baker, G. and Riser, M., 42n42
Balding, J., 190, 191n22
Baldwin, J., 186
Baldwin, J. and Wells, H., 79n13, 191n9
Baric, L., 45, 46, 47, 50
Basingstoke
  community project in, 23, 24–6
  Family Planning Association Centre in,
  162
  Family Planning Association workshops
  in, 161
  problems of, 162
Basque Government [Spain], 150
BBC [British Broadcasting Corporation],
  22, 127, 130
BEd courses, 151, 153, 154, 157
Bedworth, D. and Bedworth, A., 41n24
Belgium
  health education in, 81, 88–92, 95–6,
  220
  school health services in, 81, 88–92,
  95–6, 220
Bell, T., 31, 40n2
Bensley, L.B., Jr, 66
Bewley, B.R. *et al.*, 124n6
Black, D., 130n1
Black Report (1980), 125
Bolam, R., 191n7
'boundary issues', 83–4, 85, 211–12, 213
Bradley, C., 41n24
Bredderman, T., 133, 143

229